OXFORD MEDICAL PUBLICATIONS
Essentials of Dental Caries

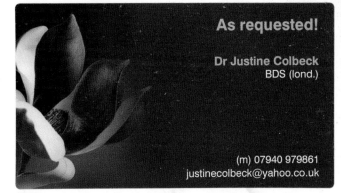

As requested!

Dr Justine Colbeck
BDS (lond.)

(m) 07940 979861
justinecolbeck@yahoo.co.uk

Essentials of Dental Caries The Disease and Its Management

Second Edition

Edwina A.M. Kidd

Professor of Cariology
United Medical and Dental School
University of London

Sally Joyston-Bechal

Honorary Senior Lecturer
St Bartholomew's and the
Royal London School
of Medicine and Dentistry
University of London

OXFORD NEW YORK TORONTO
OXFORD UNIVERSITY PRESS
1997

Oxford University Press, Walton Street, Oxford OX2 6DP

Oxford New York

Athens Auckland Bangkok Bombay
Calcutta Cape Town Dar es Salaam Delhi
Florence Hong Kong Istanbul Karachi
Kuala Lumpur Madras Madrid Melbourne
Mexico City Nairobi Paris Singapore
Taipei Tokyo Toronto
and associated companies in
Berlin Ibadan

Oxford is a trade mark of Oxford University Press

Published in the United States
by Oxford University Press Inc., New York

A catalogue record for this book is available from the British Library

Library of Congress Cataloging in Publication Data
(Data applied for)

ISBN   0 19 262692 2 Hbk
ISBN   0 19 262691 4 Pbk

Typeset by EXPO Holdings, Malaysia

Printed in Hong Kong

Preface

The first edition of this book was published by John Wright in 1987 as part of their Dental Practitioner Handbook Series. Our aim was to produce a cariology text which the junior undergraduate might find easy to read and clinically relevant. By bringing basic theoretical concepts to the chairside we hoped that the student would understand the rationale behind the clinical techniques.

The book has also been used by dental nurses, dental health educators, hygienists, and therapists. In addition, scientists working in the dental field have also found this a useful introduction to clinical cariology.

In this updated second edition, now published by Oxford University Press, we have continued to keep the text simple in the hope that the reader will be sufficiently stimulated to use this text as a springboard to the necessary further study. Indeed, there are many other comprehensive texts and this book seeks to complement them. To this end, the use of references has been kept to a minimum. Where possible, review articles or chapters in the more comprehensive texts are referred to, but where such reviews do not exist more extensive reference lists are included.

In this edition Teresa Barker has written the chapter on Patient Motivation. Mrs Barker is a dental hygienist with a degree in health psychology and many years' experience of teaching dental students.

London
June 1996   E.K.
                                                                                               S.J.B.

Acknowledgements

The manuscript was word processed by Mrs Cecilia Rodrigues, and we are grateful for her patience and care.

Contents

1

Introduction

1.1 THE CARIOUS PROCESS

The carious process affects the mineralized tissues of the teeth, namely enamel, dentine, and cementum, and is caused by the action of microorganisms on fermentable carbohydrates in the diet. It can ultimately result in demineralization of the mineral portion of these tissues followed by disintegration of the organic material. At the crystal level, initiation of the carious process may be inevitable but progression of a microscopic lesion to a clinically detectable lesion is not a certainty because in its early stages the process can be arrested and a carious lesion may become inactive. However, progression of the lesion into dentine can ultimately result in bacterial invasion and death of the pulp and spread of infection into the periapical tissues, causing pain.

1.2 AETIOLOGY OF DENTAL CARIES

Some *plaque bacteria* are capable of fermenting a suitable dietary *carbohydrate substrate* (such as the sugars sucrose and glucose) to produce acid, causing the plaque pH to fall to below 5 within one to three minutes.

Repeated falls in pH in *time* may result in the demineralization of a *susceptible site on a tooth surface*, thus initiating the carious process.

1.2.1 Dental plaque[1,2]

Dental plaque is an adherent deposit of bacteria and their products, which forms on all tooth surfaces. It is not an accidental accumulation of bacteria but develops in a sequence of steps.

When a clean enamel surface is exposed to the oral environment it becomes covered with an amorphous organic film called the pellicle. This consists mainly of a glycoprotein precipitated from saliva; it is very tenacious and can attract and help anchor specific types of bacteria to the tooth surface.

The organisms which initially colonize the pellicle are predominantly coccal in form. A large proportion of these are streptococci but only about 2 per cent of these are mutans streptococci. This is interesting because, as will be seen later, these organisms are particularly associated with initiation of the carious process. Within a few days the plaque becomes thicker and a mixture of different types of microorganisms comprise the bacterial community. Consequently, the flora of the plaque changes from its initial predominantly coccal form to a mixed flora consisting of cocci, rods, and filaments. There are local variations in the microflora at different sites on the tooth surface and these differences may explain why some sites experience a high caries activity while neighbouring sites in the same mouth remain relatively free from clinically detectable caries.

The essential role of bacteria

In a series of animal experiments in the 1950s, Orland and Keyes and co-workers showed that bacteria were essential for the production of a carious lesion. They fed rodents a highly cariogenic diet and found that they did not develop caries when kept in germ-free conditions. Caries only developed in these animals when bacteria were introduced. In 1960 Keyes infected germ-free animals with known strains of streptococci and found that these organisms were transferred to uninfected litter mates who then became susceptible to caries. He thus demonstrated that dental caries was potentially infectious and transmissible.

In order to establish which organisms were cariogenic, experiments were carried out using rodents with a known flora. (Animals with a known flora are called gnotobiotic.) This work showed that mutans streptococci and some strains of lactobacilli and actinomyces were of particular relevance to caries in these animals. Subsequently, such organisms, taken from human lesions, were used to induce caries in previously caries-free monkeys fed a high-sugar diet. It was also shown that the organisms, and consequently susceptibility to caries, could be transferred, probably by oral contact, from mother to offspring. However, adult cage-mates were more resistant, perhaps because their oral flora was already established.

Mutans streptococci and lactobacilli are cariogenic because they are able to produce acid rapidly from fermentable carbohydrates (acidogenic). They thrive under acid conditions (aciduric) and are able to adhere to the tooth surface because of their ability to synthesize sticky extracelluar polysaccharides from dietary sugars. These polysaccharides, which are mainly polymers of glucose, give the matrix of dental plaque its gelatinous consistency. Consequently, they help bacteria to stick to each other and to the tooth and, by thickening the layer of plaque, prevent saliva from neutralizing plaque acid.

1.2.2 The role of dietary carbohydrate

It is necessary for fermentable carbohydrates and plaque to be present on the tooth surface for a minimum length of time for acid to form and cause demineralization of dental enamel. These carbohydrates provide the plaque bacteria with the substrate for acid production and the synthesis of extracelluar polysaccharides. However, carbohydrates are not all equally cariogenic. While complex carbohydrates such as starch are relatively harmless because they are not completely digested in the mouth, the low molecular weight carbohydrates (sugars) diffuse readily into plaque and are metabolized quickly by the bacteria. Thus, many sugar-containing foods and drinks cause a rapid drop in plaque pH to a level which can cause demineralization of dental enamel. The plaque remains acid for some time, taking 30–60 minutes to return to its normal pH in the region of 7. The gradual return of pH to baseline values is a result of acids diffusing out of the plaque and buffers in the plaque and salivary film overlying it, exerting a neutralizing effect. *Repeated* and *frequent* consumption of sugar will keep plaque pH depressed and cause demineralization of the teeth.

The change in plaque pH may be represented graphically over a period of time following a glucose rinse (Fig. 1.1). Such a graph is called a 'Stephan curve' after the person who first described it in 1944. Once a cavity, or hole, forms in the tooth the plaque within it becomes even more efficient at producing acid. Lower pH values are recorded in plaque within cavities when compared with plaque on inactive lesions or sound surfaces in the same individuals.[3]

The synthesis of extracelluar polysaccharides from sucrose is more rapid than from glucose, fructose, and lactose. Consequently, sucrose is the most cariogenic sugar, although the other sugars are also harmful. Since sucrose is also the sugar eaten most commonly, it is a very important cause of dental caries.

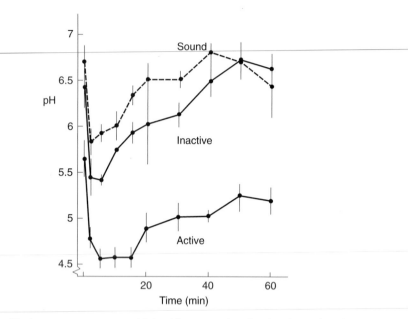

Fig. 1.1.   Stephan response curves obtained from sound occlusal surfaces, inactive occlusal carious lesions, and deep, active occlusal carious cavities following a sucrose rinse in a group of 14-year-olds. Bars indicate standard errors.[3] (Reproduced by kind permission of Professor Fejerskov.)

1.2.3 The susceptibility of the tooth surface

Tooth morphology: susceptible sites

Bacterial plaque is an essential precursor of caries, and for this reason sites on the tooth surface which favour plaque retention and stagnation are particularly prone to decay. These sites are:

1. Enamel pits and fissures on occlusal surfaces of molars and premolars (Fig. 1.2), buccal pits of molars, and palatal pits of maxillary incisors.
2. Approximal enamel smooth surfaces just cervical to the contact point (Fig. 1.3).
3. The enamel of the cervical margin of the tooth just coronal to the gingival margin (Figs 1.4a–c).
4. In patients where periodontal disease has resulted in gingival recession, the area of plaque stagnation is on the exposed root surface (Fig. 1.5).
5. The margins of restorations, particularly those that are deficient or overhanging.
6. Tooth surfaces adjacent to dentures and bridges which increase the areas where stagnation can occur.

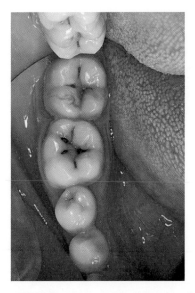

Fig. 1.2. Occlusal caries in molars, showing stained fissures. Cavities were present.

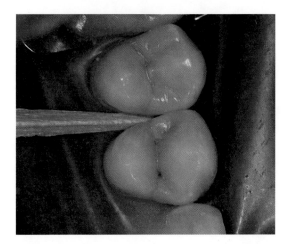

Fig. 1.3. A carious lesion is present on the distal aspect of the upper first premolar. The lesion is shining up through the marginal ridge which shows a pinkish-grey discolouration.

Environment of the tooth: saliva, and fluoride

Under normal conditions, the tooth is continually bathed in saliva. Since the susceptibility of the tooth to caries depends to a large extent on its environment, saliva has a considerable part to play (see Section 5.4). It is capable of remineralizing the early carious lesion because it is

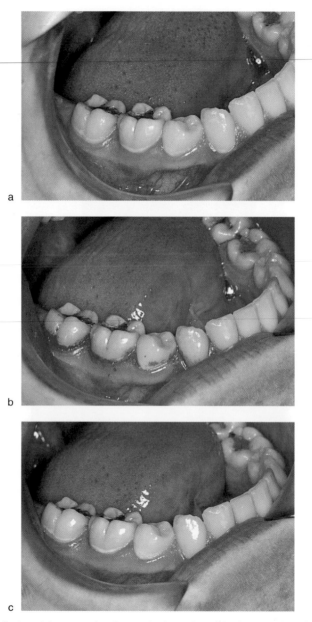

Fig. 1.4. Caries of the enamel at the cervical margins of the lower molars. (a) The white spot lesions covered with plaque. (b) A red dye has been used to stain the plaque so that the patient can see the plaque clearly. (c) The patient has now removed the stained plaque with a toothbrush; the white spot lesions are now very obvious. Note they have formed in an area of plaque stagnation and this can be shown to the patient to demonstrate the importance of plaque removal.

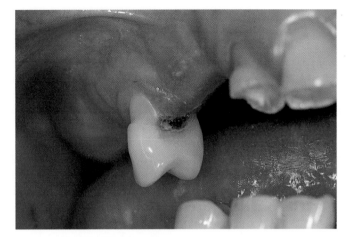

Fig. 1.5. Caries on the exposed root surface of the mesial aspect of the upper premolar. Note the lesion is in an area of plaque stagnation. Dentine is also exposed buccally but this has been cleaned and abraded by the toothbrush and is caries-free.

supersaturated with calcium and phosphate ions. This remineralizing capacity of saliva is enhanced when the fluoride ion is present. When salivary flow is diminished or absent there is increased food retention. Since salivary buffering capacity has been lost, a low pH environment is encouraged and persists longer. This in turn encourages aciduric bacteria which relish the acid conditions and continue to metabolize carbohydrate in the low pH environment. The stage is set for uncontrolled carious attack.

The presence of optimum concentrations of fluoride in the environment and in the dental tissues exerts an anticaries effect in several ways (see Section 7.3). The most important mechanism is probably its ability to retard the rate of progression of the lesion.

1.2.4 Time

The carious process consists of alternating periods of destruction and repair and the saliva has the ability to delay progression of lesions. Thus, when saliva is present, caries does not destroy the tooth in days or weeks but rather in months or years, or not at all. There is a great deal of scope to modify the carious process.

1.3 CLASSIFICATION OF DENTAL CARIES

Caries can be classified according to the anatomical site of the lesion. Thus the lesion may commence in *pits and fissures* or on *smooth surfaces*. Smooth-surface lesions may start on enamel or on the exposed root cementum and dentine *(root caries)*. Alternatively, caries may develop at the margin of a restoration. This is called *recurrent* or *secondary caries*.

Dental caries may also be classified according to the severity or rapidity of the attack. Different teeth and surfaces are involved depending on the area of plaque stagnation and the severity of the carious challenge. Thus with a mild challenge only the most vulnerable teeth and surfaces are attacked, such as the cervical margin of the teeth or the occlusal pits and fissures of permanent molars. A moderate challenge may also involve approximal surfaces of posterior teeth whereas with a severe challenge anterior teeth, which normally remain caries-free, also become carious.

Caries is a multifactorial disease. Strictly speaking its cause is pH fluctuations in bacterial plaque but these in turn may be influenced by such factors as diet, oral hygiene, salivary flow, and fluoride. In addition a number of other variables are important such as patients' knowledge of dental disease and motivation to keep their teeth. Thus patients vary in their susceptibility to the carious process and in managing dental caries, it is essential to tailor the treatment to the needs of the individual patient.

Rampant caries is the name given to a sudden rapid destruction of many teeth, frequently involving surfaces of teeth that are usually caries-free. It may be seen in the permanent dentition of teenagers and is usually due to taking frequent cariogenic snacks and sweet drinks between meals (Fig. 1.6). It is also seen in mouths where there is a sudden marked reduction in salivary flow (xerostomia) (Fig. 1.7). Radiation in the region of the salivary glands, used in the treatment of malignant tumours, is the most common cause of an acute xerostomia (see Section 5.2.2).

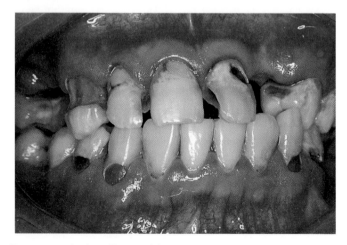

Fig. 1.6. Rampant caries in a 19-year-old man.

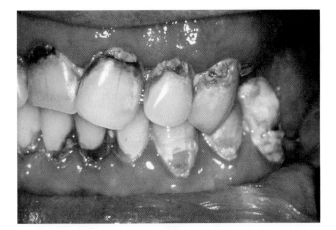

Fig. 1.7. Radiation caries. This patient had been irradiated in the region of the salivary glands for the treatment of a malignant tumour.

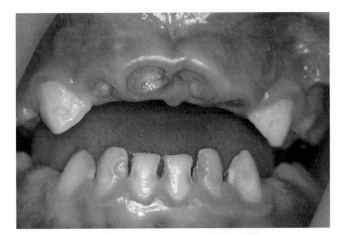

Fig. 1.8. Rampant caries of deciduous teeth. The child continually sucked a dummy filled with rose-hip syrup.

Nursing caries[4] is a particular form of rampant caries in the primary dentition of infants and young children. It is found in an infant or toddler who falls asleep sucking a bottle (called a nursing bottle) which has been filled with sweetened fluids (including milk). This bottle is given to the child in the cot before sleeping. Alternatively nursing caries may be found in infants using a pacifier dipped in sweetener or in children who have a prolonged demand breast-feeding habit. The frequency of sugar intake combined with a low salivary flow at night are important in the development of this form

of rampant caries. The clinical pattern is characteristic, with the four maxillary deciduous incisors most severely affected (Fig. 1.8).

In distinct contrast to rampant caries is *arrested caries*. This term
describes a carious lesion which does not progress. It is seen when the
oral environment has changed from conditions predisposing to caries to
conditions that tend to arrest the lesion. Figure 1.9 shows an arrested

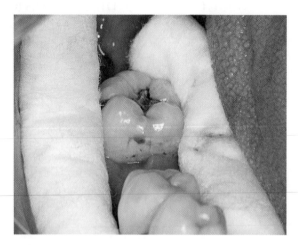

Fig. 1.9.   Arrested caries on the mesial aspect of the lower second molar. The lesion
probably stopped progressing after extraction of the lower first molar.

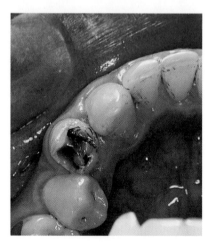

Fig. 1.10.   An arrested carious lesion in the lower first premolar. This lesion was well into
dentine, but the tissue was hard and shiny. The tooth had been in this state for at least
10 years.

lesion on the mesial aspect of a lower second molar. The lesion probably stopped progressing after extraction of the first molar. The environment changed and the surface became more easily cleaned and accessible to saliva. Figure 1.10 shows a much more advanced carious lesion which has also arrested.

1.4 EPIDEMIOLOGY OF DENTAL CARIES

Epidemiology is the study of health and disease states in populations rather than individuals. The epidemiologist defines the frequency and severity of health problems in relation to such factors as age, sex, geography, race, economic status, nutrition, and diet. It is a bird's-eye view of a problem which attempts to delineate its magnitude, study its cause, and assess the efficacy of preventive and management strategies. Epidemiological surveys are of great importance to politicians because they should indicate areas of need where public money may be appropriately spent.

1.4.1 Measuring caries activity

When studying any disease the epidemiologist is interested in both its prevalence and its incidence. Prevalence is the proportion of a population affected by a disease or condition at a particular time. Incidence is a measurement of the rate at which a disease progresses. In order to measure incidence, therefore, two examinations are required—one at the beginning and one at the end of a given time period. The incidence of the condition is then the increase or decrease in the number of new cases occurring in a population within that time period.

Before incidence and prevalence can be recorded, a quantitative measurement is required that will reflect accurately the extent of the disease in a population.

In the case of dental caries, the measurements of disease that are used are:

1. the number of decayed teeth with untreated carious lesions (D);
2. the number of teeth which have been extracted and are therefore missing (M);
3. the number of filled teeth (F).

This measurement is known as the DMF index and is an arithmetic index of the cumulative caries attack in a population. DMF(T) is used to denote decayed, missing, and filled teeth; DMF(S) denotes decayed, missing, and filled surfaces in permanent teeth and therefore takes into account the number of surfaces attacked on each tooth. The similar indices for the primary dentition are def(t) and def(s) where e denotes extracted teeth (to differentiate from loss due to natural exfoliation) and f denotes filled teeth or surfaces.

1.4.2 Practical problems in DMF and def indices

There are some potential problems in the use of these indices. In young children, missing deciduous teeth may have been lost due to natural exfoliation and these must be differentiated from those lost due to caries. Permanent teeth are lost for reasons other than caries, such as trauma, extraction for orthodontic purposes, and periodontal disease or to facilitate the construction of dentures. Third permanent molars are often removed because there is insufficient room for them in the arch. For this reason, missing teeth may be omitted from the indices and only decayed and filled surfaces included.

Epidemiologists take enormous trouble to achieve standardization of examination and recording techniques. They will practise and check their diagnoses during a clinical trial to try to ensure reproducibility. Despite this, even the trained and experienced worker will not be completely consistent on the same day, let alone consistent with others in studies spanning years.

In many populations there is a large filled component to the indices, and the dentists who have done the fillings are not standardized in their diagnosis of disease. Dentists do not practise and check their diagnostic reproducibility in the same way as epidemiologists. In addition, there is likely to be variation between dentists in their recording of disease. Epidemiologists carrying out national surveys may be limited in their access to clinical facilities because these surveys are not necessarily carried out in a dental surgery. Thus access to good lighting, the ability to clean and dry the teeth and the opportunity to examine radiographs are not available. Unless radiographs are required for clinical care it would be unethical to use ionizing radiation. Despite all these problems the indices have been, and are, of great value in assessing both the prevalence and incidence of dental caries and the effect of various preventive measures.

1.4.3 Caries prevalence in modern man[5]

Dental caries is ubiquitous in modern man and now the experience of caries is surprisingly consistent between countries, although this has not always been the situation. In the mid 1970s clinicians and research workers began to speak about a decline in the prevalence of dental caries in children. By the early 1980s data from many countries (Fig. 1.11) demonstrated this in 12-year-old children although in 1983 there were considerable intercountry differences.[6]

Nevertheless, it became clear that these secular changes in caries prevalence should have profound effects upon the pattern of practice, particularly general practice, upon dental education and upon the number and type of dental personnel required to satisfy treatment needs. Politicians naturally seized upon the good news, seeing the opportunity to spend less public money on dental services.

In the 1990s the picture that emerges worldwide is that caries prevalence has continued to decline and the similarities between countries are now marked. Figures 1.12a–d look at data from a number of countries comparing DMFT values at various ages. DMF rises with age but the consistency of the data is quite remarkable. However, a survey examination is likely to underestimate the true caries prevalence. The percentage of the

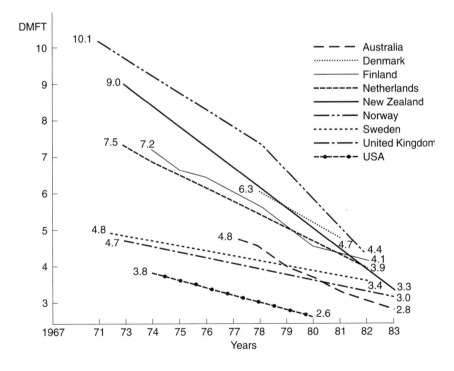

Fig. 1.11. DMFT data from 12-year-old children of many countries demonstrating a decline in caries prevalence between 1967 and 1983. Note considerable intercountry differences (source: *WHO Global Oral Data Bank* (Renson *et al.* 1986)[6]).

14

(a) Data from 12 countries providing dmft values for 5–6-year-old children in 1987–1993

Country	Year	Mean dmf	% caries free
England and Wales	1993	1.8	55
Denmark	1992	1.5	61
Finland	1991	1.4	60
Iceland	1988	2.9	40
Norway	1992	1.4	63
Sweden	1991		72
Belgium *	1990	1.05	59
Netherlands	1993	1.3	55
Switzerland	1992	1.55	
USA	1987	2.0	50
Canada	1990	1.3	65
Australia *	1992	2.0	

* 6-year-olds.

(b) Data from 14 countries providing DMFT values for 12-year-old children

Country		Year	Mean DMF	% caries free
England and Wales		1993	1.1	50
Denmark		1991	1.3	49
Finland		1991	1.2	30
Iceland		1991	2.5	23
Norway		1991	2.2	36
Sweden		1991	1.6	43
Belgium		1990	2.7	25
Germany		1993	2.5	
Netherlands				60
Eire	GHB	1992	1.5	
	WHBF	1992	1.6	
	WHB non F	1992	2.1	
Switzerland		1992	1.1	
Canada		1990	1.5	
Australia		1992	1.2	55
China (Beijing)		1993	1.3	50

(c) Data from seven studies providing DMFT values for 15-year-old children

Country	Year	Mean DMF	% caries free
England and Wales	1993	2.1	40
Denmark	1991	3.1	25
Finland	1991	3.1	23
Iceland	1991	5.3	9
Sweden	1991	3.6	70
Switzerland	1992	2.2	
Beijing	1981	2.1	29

(d) Mean DMFT values for adult dentate populations from nine countries

Country	Year	Age	Mean DMF
England and Wales	1988	35–44	19.0
Denmark	1990	30–39	17.8
Finland	1986	28	16.7
Norway	1993	35	25.0
Sweden	1985	30	17.5
Netherlands	1986	35–44	17.4
		45–54	18.4
Germany	1989	35–44	16.7
		45–54	18.4
Australia	1987/88	35–44	18.8
New Zealand	1988	35–44	18.3

Fig. 1.12. (Reproduced by kind permission of the *International Dental Journal*[6].)

population 'caries-free' should be interpreted with great care. By 'caries-free' the epidemiologist really means 'cavity-free' or free of caries in dentine. This diagnosis is usually made without the benefit of radiographs. As will be seen in Chapter 4, radiographs are extremely important in the diagnosis of dental decay and large cavities can be missed by a clinical examination alone. Careful cleaning and drying of teeth will make a clinical examination more accurate but these facilities may not be available under national survey conditions. Taking the data from present-day 15-year-old and middle-aged adults the salient question for the politician and the profession is *'will the present 15-year-old deteriorate by 15 DMFT in 25 years, or will the low caries experience of present-day teenagers ensure a much healthier dentate population when they reach middle age?'* This question can only be answered if epidemiological surveys continue.

The consistent worldwide picture of DMF values is matched by a consistency in the rate of decline in caries prevalence. Figure 1.13 shows graphs of caries experience of children in England and Wales but they serve to typify a worldwide situation.[7] Declining caries prevalence bottomed out in the 5-year-olds in the early 1980s and there is now some evidence of a rise. In the 12- and 14-year-olds the rate of decline has slowed and again there is evidence of bottoming out.

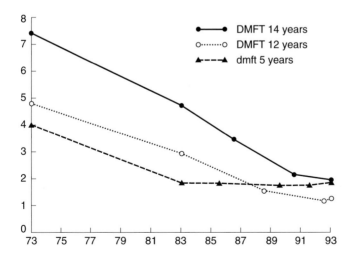

Fig. 1.13. Time trends in caries experience of children in England and Wales between 1973 and 1993. (Reproduced by kind permission of the *International Dental Journal.*[7])

1.4.4 Why has caries prevalence declined?

The reasons for the decline in caries prevalence are not fully understood. The following factors may be important:

1. The increased exposure to fluoride in water, in toothpaste, in mouthrinses, and in topical applications in the dental surgery may be of particular importance. The fluoride ion is thought to reduce the incidence of caries in several different ways (see Section 7.3).
2. An improved level of oral heath care might influence the disease. Such factors as regular visits to the dentist, improved oral hygiene, and increased awareness of the relevance of diet could all be important.
3. A changing pattern of sugar consumption could also be relevant, although there is little evidence that the per capita consumption of sucrose in the industrialized countries has fallen. This highlights the multifactorial nature of dental caries. The increased use of sugar substitutes may be important. These substances impart sweetness but cannot be fermented to acid by bacteria.
4. A decrease in virulence of the organisms may be relevant.Virulence might increase again and thus the prevalence of the disease might increase. It is also possible that the increased use of antibiotics may have affected the causative organisms.

Finding the reasons for any improvement is of more then just academic interest. Until the profession knows why this change has occurred, it will be difficult to predict future patterns. Will the caries rate continue to decrease, stay static, or increase again? If the profession has done something right it needs to be identified and continued! In addition, a knowledge of future patterns of disease has important implications for the planning of dental services for patients.

1.4.5 Skewed distribution

Although the consistency of the data is fascinating and important information, it is essential to realize that at the level of the individual patient arithmetic means are meaningless! People vary in their susceptibility to the carious process. There is evidence of this in Fig. 1.12c. Epidemiologists in Sweden claim that 70 per cent of the 15-year-old population is 'caries-free' even though this country had one of the highest mean DMFs at 3.6. This suggests that in Sweden most of the caries is concentrated in 30 per cent of the population. Sadly, in many industrialized countries the problem is now mainly concentrated in those of low socio-economic status. As far as the dentist in the surgery is concerned it is essential to identify those at risk to progressive carious attack so that preventive measures may be targeted appropriately. This important topic of caries-risk assessment will be addressed in Chapter 4.

1.5 MODIFYING THE CARIOUS PROCESS

Appreciation of the factors involved in the carious process is essential to understanding how it can be modified. It is important to regard caries as an alternating process of destruction and repair (Fig. 1.14). When the destructive forces outweigh the reparative powers of the saliva the process will progress (Chapter 5). Conversely, if the reparative forces outweigh the destructive forces, the process will arrest or even reverse, provided it is caught in its early stages. Consequently, early diagnosis is of paramount importance (Chapter 4) because if destruction is allowed to proceed too far, only operative intervention can replace the tissue (Chapter 11). Unfortunately, fillings do not prevent caries and new lesions can develop adjacent to restorations (Section 11.7). If fillings are to last, preventive treatment must go hand in hand with operative treatment.

The basis of preventive treatment is modification of one or more of the factors involved in the aetiology of the disease. Since the carious process usually takes months or years to destroy the tooth, time is on the patient's side. Theoretically there are a number of ways of modifying the carious process:

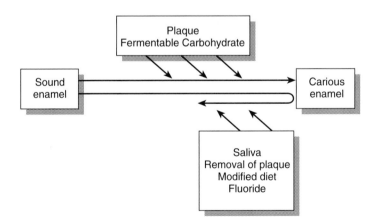

Fig. 1.14. A diagrammatic representation of the carious process as an alternating process of destruction and repair. Sound enamel will become carious in time if plaque bacteria are given the substrate they need to produce acid. However, progression of lesions can be arrested and the arrow can even be turned around towards sound enamel again by modifying diet, improving plaque control, and using fluoride appropriately.

1. *Dietary advice*. Fortunately, complete elimination of refined carbohy-drate from the diet is not necessary for the prevention of clinically detectable carious lesions, but relatively simple measures, such as reducing the frequency of consumption of sugar and confining it to mealtimes, are usually sufficient (Chapter 6). This is the most effective way of preventing caries.

2. *Oral hygiene instruction*. Demineralization occurs in areas of plaque stag-nation and thus plaque removal is extremely important in the control of the carious process (Chapter 8).

3. *Appropriate use of fluoride*. The availability of low concentrations of fluoride in drinking water, toothpaste, and mouthwashes will delay the progression of lesion (Chapter 7).

4. *Use of fissure sealants*. Deep pits and fissures can be made less suscepti-ble by obliterating or 'sealing' them with a resin (Chapter 10).

5. *Chemical plaque control*. This final arrow in the quiver may be used in high-risk patients such as those with dry mouths who are highly sus-ceptible to rampant caries through lack of saliva (Chapter 8).

It is salutary to note that each of these preventive measures requires the patient's active cooperation. The principle role of the profession, therefore, may be to provide patients with knowledge so that they understand their essential role in this control. In addition, patients need to be persuaded to accept responsibility for their own mouths (Chapter 9).

However, before discussing the management of dental caries the process itself must be understood. The following chapters describe caries in enamel and dentine and are part of the scientific basis on which management strategies rest.

REFERENCES

1. Thylstrup, A. and Fejerskov, O. (1994). *Textbook of clinical cariology*, (2nd edn), Ch. 3: Oral ecology and dental caries. Munksgaard, Copenhagen.
2. Thylstrup, A. and Fejerskov, O. (1994). *Textbook of cinical cariology*, (2nd edn), Ch. 5: Development, structure and pH of dental plaque. Munksgaard, Copenhagen.
3. Fejerskov, O., Scheie, A., and Manji, F. (1992). The effect of sucrose on plaque pH in the primary and permanent dentition of caries in active and inactive Kenyan children. *J. Dent. Res.*, **71**, 25–31.
4. Johnston, T. and Messer, L.B. (1994). Nursing caries: Literature review and report of a case managed under local anaesthesia. *Aust. Dent. J.*, **39**, 373–81.
5. Murray, J.J. (1994). Comments on the results reported at the Second International Conference 'Changes in Caries Prevalence.' *Int. Dent. J.*, **44**, 457–8.
6. Renson, C.E. (1986). Changing patterns of dental caries: a survey on 20 countries. *Ann. Acad. Med. Singapore*, **15**, 284–98.
7. Downer, M.C. (1994). Caries prevalence in the UK. *Int. Dent. J.*, **44**, 365–70.

2

Caries in enamel

2.1 BASIC ENAMEL STRUCTURE

Sound enamel consists of crystals of hydroxyapatite packed tightly together in an orderly arrangement. The crystals are so tightly packed that the enamel has a glass-like appearance but is translucent allowing the colour of the dentine to shine through it. Even though crystal packing is very tight, each crystal is actually separated from its neighbours by tiny intercrystalline spaces or pores. These spaces are filled with water and organic material. When enamel is exposed to acids produced by dental plaque, mineral is removed from the surface of the crystal which shrinks in size. Thus, the intercrystalline spaces enlarge and the tissue becomes more porous. This increase in porosity can be seen clinically.

2.2 MACROSCOPIC FEATURES OF THE 'EARLY' ENAMEL LESION

The earliest macroscopic evidence of enamel caries is known as the 'white spot lesion'. It is best seen on dried, extracted teeth where the lesion appears as a small, opaque, white area cervical to the contact point. The colour of the lesion distinguishes it from the adjacent translucent sound enamel. The colour change is based on the increased porosity of the tissue which alters the way in which the light is scattered. Enamel has a refractive index of 1.62 while the refractive index of water is 1.33. Air-drying removes the water from the intercrystalline spaces which are now filled with air, refractive index 1.0. It is these differences in refractive index which alter the scattering of the light. If air-drying reveals a white spot in the enamel, the change in enamel porosity is slight. However, if the porosity is visible as a white spot without air-drying, the porosity is larger. Thus the clinician, using vision alone, can estimate the degree of mineral loss. At this stage mineral loss cannot be detected with a probe because the enamel is hard and no cavity is present. Sometimes this lesion may appear brown in colour due to exogenous material absorbed into its porosities (Fig. 2.1).

Both white and brown spot lesions may be present in the mouth for some years because it is not inevitable for a carious lesion to progress. Figures 1.9 (see p. 10) and 2.2 are both examples of lesions which have probably been present for many years and are now static, or 'arrested'. In Fig. 1.9 the lesion on the approximal aspect of the second lower molar probably arrested after the first molar was extracted. The area became more accessible to saliva and the toothbrush so that conditions did not favour lesion progression. In Fig. 2.2 buccal lesions are present. It is likely that these lesions developed soon after the eruption of the tooth in an area of plaque stagnation near the gingival margin. However, the gingival tissues are now positioned closer to the enamel–dentine junction following passive eruption

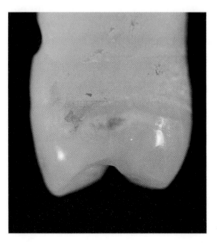

Fig. 2.1.   A carious lesion in enamel on the approximal surface of an upper premolar. This lesion is not detectable with a probe but its colour (white and brown) distinguishes it from the adjacent sound enamel.

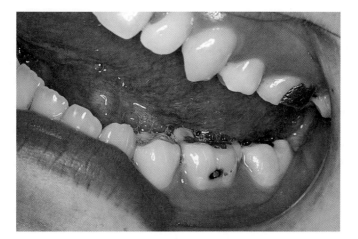

Fig. 2.2. Arrested lesions on the buccal aspect of the lower first molar. A small amalgam restoration is also present.

of the tooth. The lesions are now easily accessible for cleaning and are not progressing.

The fact that in its early stages the carious lesion can be arrested implies that efforts should be directed towards early diagnosis and prevention of further demineralization. However, if the early enamel lesion progresses, the intact surface breaks down (cavitation) and a hole is formed (a cavity).

2.3 MICROSCOPIC FEATURES OF THE 'EARLY' ENAMEL LESION

Histological studies have played an important part in the realization that dental caries is not simply a process of progressive demineralization but that removal of plaque will result in lesion arrest and even partial repair by redeposition of dissolved mineral within the lesion. This is the scientific base for the preventive treatment of the carious process.

2.3.1 Initial surface dissolution

Clinical studies, where bands have been placed on teeth to create stagnation areas, show that after a week of undisturbed plaque accumulation there are microscopic signs of direct dissolution of the outer enamel surface. However, even after careful air-drying, this cannot be seen by the clinician but only found by using a scanning electron microscope. After 14 days this surface dissolution is more obvious microscopically but now there is a tendency for preferential removal of mineral from the enamel deep to the outer surface. At this stage air-drying will reveal the white spot lesion clinically. After 4 weeks these macroscopic changes may be seen without air-drying. Clinically this active lesion would be similar to that in Fig. 1.4 (see p. 6) with a characteristic chalky or matt surface. The lack of lustre is due to direct surface loss of tissue and the white appearance to the internal enamel porosity. It is very important that clinician and patient appreciate that thorough, daily, plaque removal at this stage will arrest the lesion and indeed clinically the lesion may appear to partially heal. The sequence of events is as follows: after two to three weeks of daily plaque removal the surface will appear hard and shiny again and the white spot lesion will be less obvious. The shiny, hard, appearance is the result of abrasion or polishing of the dull, partly dissolved, surface of the active lesion. Re-precipitation of mineral occurs within the depth of the lesion and the white area becomes less obvious, and, if caught early, may even disappear.

2.3.2 Light microscope appearance of the white spot lesion on a smooth surface

The demineralization within the enamel can be seen by examining a ground section in the light microscope. These sections are cut with a diamond wheel and are then made thinner by grinding on a flat glass surface in a slurry of alumina powder and water. Once a section has been reduced to 100 μm (1000 μm = 1 mm) it is ready to be examined by transmitted light. Although plain transmitted light can be used, polarized light is often preferred because the lesion is seen clearly.

On a smooth surface, such as the approximal or buccal, the lesion is usually cone shaped, the apex of the cone pointing towards the enamel–dentine junction (Fig. 2.3a). The lesion is this shape because it follows the direction of the enamel prisms. The centre of the cone corresponds to the deepest portion of the lesion and is the oldest and most active part of the lesion. The enamel lesion spreads laterally on the surface of the tooth as new lesions are generated by the growth and evolution of cariogenic plaque.

The small lesion has been divided into zones based upon its histological appearance when longitudinal ground sections are examined with the light microscope. Four zones may be distinguished. There is a *translucent zone* at the inner advancing front of the lesion, while a *dark zone* may be found just superficial to this. The *body of the lesion* is the third zone lying between the dark zone and the apparently undamaged surface enamel. This zone makes up the major part of the lesion and shows the most marked demineralization. The relatively unaffected *surface zone* superficial to the lesion is the

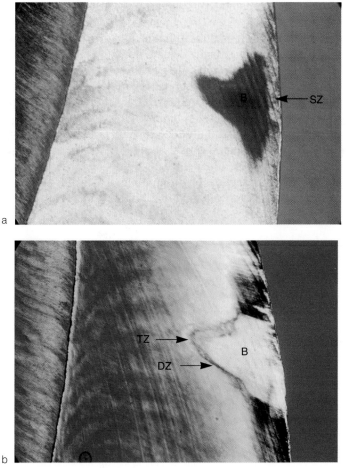

Fig. 2.3. (a) Longitudinal ground section through a small lesion of enamel caries on a smooth surface examined in water with polarized light. The lesion is cone shaped. The body of the lesion (B) appears dark beneath a relatively intact surface zone (SZ). (Magnification ×135). (b) The same section as in (a) now examined in quinoline with the polarizing microscope. A translucent zone (TZ) is present at the advancing front of the lesion and a dark zone (DZ) can be seen superficial to this. The body (B) of the lesion appears translucent. (Magnification ×135.)

fourth zone. The appearance of each of these four zones of enamel caries in polarized light will now be described.

Zone 1: the translucent zone

The translucent zone of enamel caries is not seen in all lesions but when it is present it lies at the advancing front of the lesion and is the first recognizable alteration from normal enamel. This zone is only seen when a longitudinal ground section is examined in a clearing agent, such as quinoline, having the same refractive index (1.62) as that of enamel. The translucent zone appears structureless, the translucency being demarcated from normal enamel on its deep aspect and the dark zone on its superficial aspect (Fig. 2.3b).

The translucent zone is a more porous region than sound enamel, the pores having been created by the demineralization process. Sound enamel has a pore volume of about 0.1 per cent. The translucent zone, however, has a pore volume of approximately 1 per cent. The pores are probably located at junctional sites such as prism borders, cross striations, and along striae of Retzius. Once these areas fill with quinoline structural markings are lost, due to the penetration of the quinoline which has an identical refractive index to that of enamel apatite. This is why the translucent zone looks translucent.

Zone 2: the dark zone

If a translucent zone is present at the advancing front of a lesion when examined in quinoline, the dark zone is the second zone of alteration from normal enamel and lies just superficial to the translucent zone. The zone appears dark when the ground section is placed in quinoline (Fig. 2.3b).

The dark zone is more porous than the translucent zone, having a pore volume of 2–4 per cent. The evidence explaining why the dark zone appears dark is intriguing. It would seem that in this zone the pores are of varying sizes, large and small. Quinoline is a large molecule and cannot enter the small pores which remain filled with air, giving a dark appearance.

Theoretically there are two ways in which these small pores may have formed. They may have been created by demineralization, that is by an opening up of sites not previously attacked. Alternatively, the small pores could represent areas of repair where mineral has been redeposited. There is now considerable evidence to support the view that the dark zone can represent an area of redeposition of mineral. If arrested lesions, which have been present clinically for many years, are examined histologically, they show wide, well developed dark zones at the front of the lesion, within the body of the lesion and at the surface of the lesion (Fig. 2.4).

Zone 3: the body of the lesion

The body of the lesion comprises the largest proportion of carious enamel in the small lesion. It lies superficial to the dark zone and deep to the relatively unaffected surface layer of the lesion. When a longitudinal ground section is examined in quinoline in polarized light, the area appears translucent and the striae of Retzius may be well marked (Fig. 2.3b).

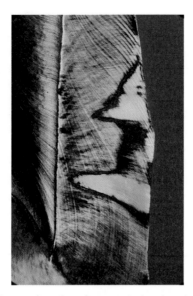

Fig. 2.4. Longitudinal ground section of an arrested carious lesion in a tooth extracted from a patient aged 65 years. The section is examined in quinoline with polarized light and shows wide, well developed dark zones at the advancing front of the lesion, within the body of the lesion and at the surface of the lesion. (Magnification x135.)

The body of the lesion is seen particularly clearly if the ground section is examined in water (Fig. 2.3a). The water molecules enter the pores in the tissue, and since the refractive index of water is different to that of enamel, the area appears dark. The pore volume of this region is 5 per cent at its periphery, increasing to 25 per cent or more in the centre.

Zone 4: the surface zone

One of the important characteristics of enamel caries is that the small lesion remains covered by a surface layer which appears relatively unaffected by the attack although, as discussed earlier, in the active lesion there is direct dissolution of this outermost surface. The zone is most clearly seen in polarized light when the section is in water where it appears as a relatively unaffected area superficial to the body of the lesion (Fig. 2.3a). The zone has a pore volume of approximately 1 per cent, but if the lesion progresses the surface layer is eventually destroyed and a cavity forms.

The subsurface demineralization that characterizes the 'early' enamel lesion has intrigued research workers for many years and is still not fully understood. Some have suggested that the formation of this relatively unaffected surface layer is associated with the special properties of surface enamel which shows a high degree of mineralization, a higher fluoride content, and possibly a greater amount of insoluble protein than subsurface enamel. However, a surface zone can also be produced when the original enamel surface has been ground away. Consequently the existence of surface enamel with 'special' characteristics cannot be entirely responsible.

Another explanation for the relative protection of this outermost enamel, which is next to the pellicle and plaque, must be the dynamic processes taking place at this interface. The chemical explanation is as follows: when the pH of the plaque fluid drops to below 5.5, hydroxyapatite may dissolve and fluorapatite may form in the demineralized surface enamel. Thus, destruction (demineralization) and repair (remineralization) are a part of the carious process. The principal action of fluoride is to favour this repair.

2.3.3 Light microscope appearance of occlusal caries

Occlusal fissures and buccal pits can be stagnation areas where plaque may form and mature, protected from functional wear and access to a toothbrush.

The histological features of fissures caries are similar to those already described for smooth surfaces. The lesion forms around the fissure walls (Fig. 2.5). Eventually the lesions increase in size, coalescing at the base of the fissure. The enamel lesion broadens as it approaches the underlying

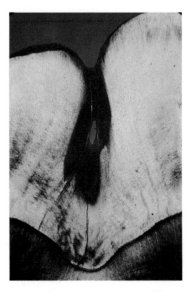

Fig. 2.5.   A longitudinal ground section through an occlusal fissure showing a small carious lesion. The section is in water and viewed in polarized light. The lesion forms on the fissure walls giving the appearance of two smooth surface lesions. (Magnification x 90.)

dentine, guided by prism direction. Thus the lesion assumes the shape of a cone with its base towards the enamel–dentine junction. This explains why a small cavity on an occlusal surface may apparently conceal a large lesion in dentine.

2.3.4 Enamel lesions in deciduous teeth

The histological features of enamel caries in deciduous teeth are similar to those already described in permanent enamel. However, the enamel in deciduous teeth is much thinner than in permanent teeth and the pulps are relatively large. For this reason early diagnosis of caries in deciduous enamel is of particular importance.

2.3.5 Microradiography

In the laboratory it is possible to take a radiograph of a ground section. This is called a microradiograph and it may be examined in the light microscope. The technique will demonstrate demineralization in excess of 5 per cent as a radiolucent area (Fig. 2.6) which corresponds almost exactly with the body of the lesion as seen in polarized light when the section is in water. A well mineralized radio-opaque surface layer is apparent.

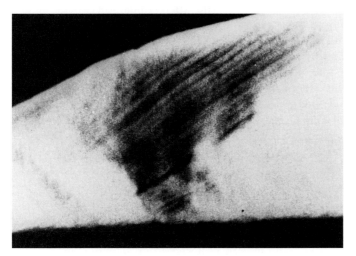

Fig. 2.6.   A microradiograph of a ground section showing a carious lesion in the enamel. The body of the lesion shows marked radiolucency and the striae of Retzius can be seen clearly. Superficially the surface of the enamel appears well mineralized. (Magnification x90.)

2.4 THE MICROBIOLOGY OF ENAMEL CARIES

The carious process can be initiated by a normal oral flora. However, after a few days the acid environment of the lesion favours colonization with aciduric microorganisms such as mutans streptococci and lactobacilli. Thus, as conditions change in the area of the lesion, there are ecological shifts in the microflora.

Longitudinal studies on the succession of bacterial populations in plaque as a lesion develops show that different waves of microorganisms may be involved during different stages of lesion development. While mutans streptococci are associated with early demineralization, lactobacilli appear to be related to lesion progression. These cariogenic bacteria have the distinctive ability to transport sugars and convert them rapidly to acid, even under extremely low pH. Few oral bacteria are able to survive and multiply in such acidic conditions.

Although there is no doubt that mutans streptococci and lactobacilli are the most important microorganisms implicated in caries, the microbial ecology of the mouth is highly complex. In some cases caries can develop in their apparent absence and they can also be harboured without evidence of caries.

2.5 LESION ARREST

It is very important to realize that the carious process can be arrested by simple clinical measures such as improved plaque control, altered diet, and sensible use of fluoride. It is therefore the clinician's responsibility to detect enamel caries in its earliest form by careful visual inspection of teeth after cleaning and drying. The clinician can now help the patient tip the balance in favour of lesion arrest rather than lesion progression. An arrested white spot lesion is more resistant to acid attack than sound enamel. It may be regarded as scar tissue and should not be attacked with a dental drill.

2.6 CAVITATION

If, on the other hand, the lesion progresses, the surface zone eventually breaks down and a cavity forms (Figs 2.7a and b). Plaque now forms within the cavity and may be protected from cleaning aids such as a toothbrush filament or dental floss. For this reason a cavitated lesion is more likely to progress, although it can still arrest if it is on a surface which is accessible to a toothbrush and diet is changed.

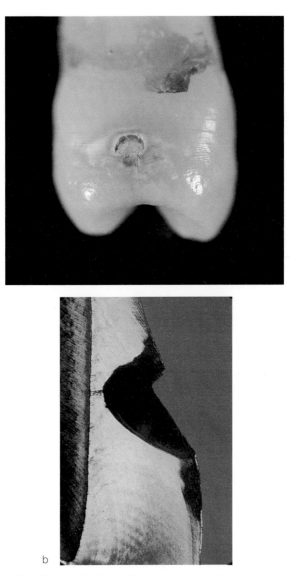

Fig. 2.7.   a. A cavitated enamel lesion on the approximal surface of a premolar tooth. b. A longitudinal ground section through this lesion examined in water with the polarizing microscope.

REFERENCE

Thylstrup, A. and Fejerskov, O. (1994). *Textbook of clinical cariology*, (2nd edn), Ch. 6, Clinical and pathological features of dental caries. Munksgaard, Copenhagen.

3

Caries in dentine and its effect on the pulp

3.1 SHAPE OF LESIONS: SMOOTH SURFACE AND FISSURE

It has been emphasized in Chapter 2 that enamel carious lesions on smooth surfaces and in fissures differ in shape because of the anatomy of the fissure and the direction of the enamel prisms. The smooth surface lesion is cone shaped, the base of the cone being at the enamel surface. The fissure lesion is also ultimately cone shaped but the base of the cone is at the enamel–dentine junction. This is because the spread of the enamel lesion is guided by prism direction and hence the fissure lesion broadens as it approaches the dentine.

When and if the carious process reaches the enamel–dentine junction, caries appears to spread laterally along the junction to involve the dentine on a wider front. Sound enamel appears to be undermined by the carious process in dentine and the resulting lesion is larger than would be expected from examination of the enamel alone, particularly in fissure lesions (Figs 3.1

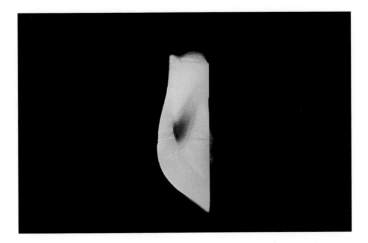

Fig. 3.1. A hemisection of an approximal carious lesion. Note the apparent lateral spread of caries along the enamel–dentine junction. In dentine the carious process follows the dentinal tubules.

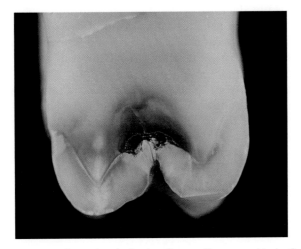

Fig. 3.2. A hemisection of a carious lesion in a fissure. The enamel lesion has formed on the walls of the fissure. There is extensive undermining of the enamel. The clinical appearance of this lesion was similar to Fig. 1.2.

and 3.2). However, it has recently been claimed that this apparent lateral spread is in fact the response of the dentine to events taking place in the enamel directly above it. Nevertheless, clinically the enamel appears to be undermined and brittle and may eventually fracture under occlusal forces to produce a large cavity. The apparent undermining of enamel by the carious process is of relevance in cavity preparation because enamel must often be removed to gain access to the soft and infected carious dentine beneath it.

3.2 THE PULP–DENTINE COMPLEX

The carious process in enamel is mainly dependent on inorganic chemical reactions but caries in dentine involves living tissues. Dentine is a vital tissue containing the cytoplasmic extensions of the odontoblasts in the dentinal tubules. The odontoblast cell bodies line the pulp chamber and their continued vitality is dependent on the blood supply and lymphatic drainage of the pulp tissue. Thus dentine must be considered together with pulp since the two tissues are so intimately connected. The pulp–dentine complex, like any other vital tissue in the body, is capable of defending itself. The state of the tissue at any time will depend on the state of the balance between the attacking forces and the defence reactions.

3.3 POTENTIAL CAUSES OF PULPAL INJURY

Dental caries is not the only cause of pulpal injury; however, the defence reactions of the tissue are the same irrespective of the stimulus. The stimuli which may invoke the defence reactions include *bacteria* as in dental caries, and *mechanical* stimuli, such as trauma, tooth fracture, cavity preparation, and tooth wear. In addition, *chemical* stimuli are important, for example, acids in foods, toxic dental restorative materials, and dehydration of dentine which is particularly likely during cavity preparation. Finally, *thermal* shocks, such as excess heat generated by careless use of rotary instruments during cavity preparation or temperature changes transmitted to dentine through large metal restorations from hot or cold foods can be damaging.

3.4 DEFENCE REACTIONS OF THE PULP–DENTINE COMPLEX

The following defence reactions are of importance:

- tubular sclerosis within the dentine
- reactionary dentine at the interface between dentine and pulp
- inflammation of the pulp.

Note that all these defence reactions depend on the presence of a vital pulp.

3.4.1 Tubular sclerosis

Tubular sclerosis (Fig. 3.3) is a process in which mineral is deposited within the lumina of the dentinal tubules and may be thought of as an extension of the normal mechanism of peritubular dentine formation.

The response, which requires the action of vital odontoblasts, is commonly seen at the periphery of carious lesions in dentine. Tubular sclerosis results in the affected area being structurally more homogeneous. For this reason there is less scattering of light as it passes through the tissue and the area of dentine is called a *translucent zone*. The term 'translucent zone' should not be confused with the translucent zone of enamel caries. In the enamel lesion the translucent zone represents demineralization whereas in the dentine lesion it represents increased mineral content!

Tubular sclerosis may be protective in that it reduces the permeability of the tissue, thus potentially inhibiting the penetration of acids and bacterial toxins.

3.4.2 Reactionary dentine

Reactionary or reparative dentine (Fig. 3.4) is a layer of dentine formed at the interface between the dentine and pulp. It is formed in response to a

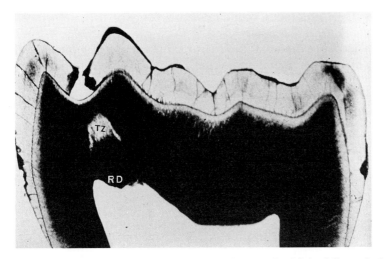

Fig. 3.3. A ground section of a molar crown viewed in transmitted light. A fissure lesion is present. The enamel is cavitated. Tubular sclerosis is seen as a translucent zone in the dentine (TZ). Reactionary dentine (RD) is also present since the pulp horn is partially obliterated. (By courtesy of Professor N.W. Johnson.)

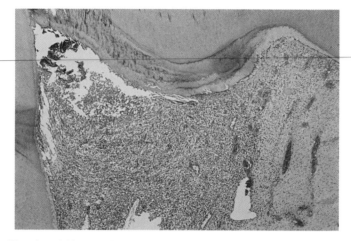

Fig. 3.4. Chronic pulpitis as indicated by the reactionary dentine formation. A predominantly chronic (mononuclear) inflammatory infiltrate is gradually extending across and has largely replaced the normal coronal pulp tissue. (By courtesy of Professor R. Cawson.)

stimulus acting further peripherally and for this reason its distribution is limited to the area beneath the stimulus.

Reactionary dentine should be distinguished from primary dentine which is formed before tooth eruption and secondary dentine which forms throughout life.

Reactionary dentine varies in structure from a well formed tissue with evenly placed tubules indistinguishable from the adjacent primary and secondary dentine, through varying degrees of irregularity in the tubules and degrees of mineralization, to an abnormally formed tissue with few tubules and numerous interglobular areas and even entrapped odontoblasts.

Regular reactionary dentine forms in response to a mild stimulus but with increasing severity of the stimulus there is increasing likelihood of damage to the odontoblasts and dysplasia of the reactionary tissue formed. An overwhelming stimulus can result in death of the odontoblasts and, in this case, no reactionary dentine will be formed. However, sometimes other cells in the pulp differentiate to form an atubular calcified material.

It is thought that the blood supply to the pulp is an important factor determining its ability to produce reactionary dentine. Reactionary dentine may not be formed if the blood supply is poor and it has been suggested that young teeth may form reactionary dentine more readily than old teeth for this reason. In addition, the severity of the stimulus may be relevant. A slowly progressing, small lesion may give time for a considerable reparative dentine response whereas with a more rapidly progressing lesion the response may be disorganized or even non-existent.

When formed, reactionary dentine provides extra protection for the odontoblasts and other cells of the pulp by increasing the distance between them and the injurious stimulus. In rather simple terms the pulp can be considered to be 'running away' and its retreat has important implications in the operative management of caries, as will be seen in Chapter 11.

3.4.3 Inflammation of the pulp

Inflammation is the fundamental response of all vascular connective tissues to injury. Inflammation of the pulp is called *pulpitis* and, as in any other tissue, it may be acute or chronic. The duration and intensity of the stimulus is partly responsible for the type of response. A low-grade, long-lasting stimulus may result in chronic inflammation whereas a sudden, severe stimulus is more likely to provoke an acute pulpitis.

In a slowly progressing carious lesion in dentine, the stimuli reaching the pulp are bacterial toxins and thermal and osmotic shocks from the external environment. The response to these low-grade, sustained stimuli is chronic inflammation which is well localized beneath the cavity. One rationale for restoring a cavity in a tooth is to remove the soft, infected dentine which is acting as an irritant and fill the cavity with a restoration. The local inflammation then has the potential to repair. However, if the carious process continues, the organisms actually reach the pulp to create a 'carious exposure', and now localized acute inflammation is likely to supervene and be superimposed on the chronic inflammation.

Inflammatory reactions have vascular and cellular components. The cellular component is most obvious in chronic inflammation (Fig. 3.4) with lymphocytes, plasma cells, monocytes, and macrophages all present within the tissue. In time there may be increased collagen production leading to fibrosis. These chronic inflammatory reactions may not endanger the vitality of the tooth.

Unfortunately, the same cannot be said of acute inflammation, since in this process the vascular changes predominate, including dilatation of blood vessels, producing an initial acceleration of blood flow and fluid exudate. This exudate may later result in retardation of blood flow and vascular stasis. There is active emigration of neutrophils (Fig. 3.5) and all these factors contribute to an increase in tension of the tissue.

The outcome of this process is often localized necrosis, and in time this may involve the entire pulp. The sequel to pulpal necrosis is spread of inflammation into the periapical tissues (apical periodontitis). Once again, the inflammatory response may be acute or chronic.

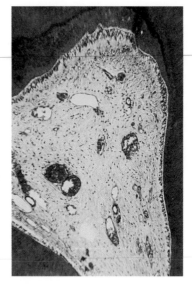

Fig. 3.5. Early acute pulpitis showing the widely dilated pulp vessels and early emigration of leucocytes. There is patchy oedema of the dying odontoblast layer. (By courtesy of Professor R. Cawson.)

3.4.4 Symptoms of pulpitis

Many studies have attempted to correlate the symptoms of which a patient complains with the level of inflammation in the pulp as determined by histological examination. These correlations are poor and for this reason it is only possible to make some generalizations relating a patient's symptoms to the histological condition of the pulp.

The first of these generalizations is that a chronically inflamed pulp is usually symptomless. In contrast, acute inflammation is almost always painful, the painful response being initiated by hot, cold, or sweet stimuli. Unfortunately the pain is often not well localized to the offending tooth and the patient may not be able to indicate which quadrant, or even which side of the mouth, is involved.

What matters to the clinician is whether or not the pulp is likely to survive, as a pulp that will die should be removed and the pulp canal sealed with an inert filling material (root canal filling) or the tooth should be extracted. Since clinical symptoms relate so poorly to pulp pathology there is an obvious problem here. A useful rule of thumb is to divide clinical pulpitis into *reversible pulpitis* and *irreversible pulpitis*.

In reversible pulpitis the clinician hopes to be able to preserve a healthy vital pulp. The clinical diagnosis of reversible pulpitis is made when the pain evoked by a hot, cold, or sweet stimulus is of short duration, disappearing when the stimulus is removed. On the other hand, if pain persists for minutes or hours after removal of the stimulus, a clinical diagnosis of irreversible pulpitis may be made and the pulp removed and replaced by a root filling. Alternatively, the tooth may be extracted.

Whereas acutely inflamed pulps are painful, necrotic pulps are painless since there are no viable nerves to transmit pain. However, once the periapical tissues are involved, another set of symptoms may develop. Chronic periapical inflammation is usually painless, but acute periapical inflammation is often very uncomfortable, the pain being well localized. The inflammatory exudate is sometimes sufficient to raise the tooth slightly in the socket. Such a tooth is tender to bite on and tender to touch because it acts as a piston in its socket transmitting forces directly to the inflamed periapical tissues. It is possible for acute periapical inflammation to become chronic and for chronic inflammation to become acute. The inflammation from acute periodontitis can spread to the adjacent soft tissues and produce a dramatic swelling. Eventually pus may discharge through a sinus and at this point pain is relieved and inflammation may then become chronic.

3.5 HISTOLOGICAL APPEARANCES: DEGENERATIVE AND DESTRUCTIVE CHANGES

The appearance of a carious lesion in dentine depends on the balance reached between the defence reactions already described and the destructive processes. The destructive processes include:

- demineralization of dentine
- destruction of the organic matrix
- damage and death of the odontoblast
- pulpal inflammation proceeding to necrosis.

The pulp–dentine complex will respond to the carious challenge before cavitation of the enamel, that is while the microorganisms are still confined to the tooth surface. This is particularly obvious in a slowly progressing lesion.

Once there is cavitation of enamel, bacteria can reach the dentine. These bacteria receive more protection than those on the surface of the tooth and these conditions favour an ecological shift in the population of bacteria towards anaerobic and acid-producing bacteria. At this stage the spectrum of defence reactions will be seen together with more marked destructive or degenerative changes.

3.5.1 Histological appearance of the lesion before cavitation of the enamel

Figure 3.6 is a diagrammatic representation of a carious lesion developing on a smooth enamel surface. The four zones of enamel caries can be seen (translucent zone, dark zone, body of lesion, and surface zone). The advancing front of the enamel lesion has reached the enamel–dentine junction but the enamel surface is still intact. However, since the carious enamel is porous, acids, enzymes, and other chemical stimuli from the tooth surface will reach the outer dentine evoking a response in the pulp–dentine complex. The defence reactions of reactionary dentine and translucent dentine may be seen, together with some demineralization near the enamel–dentine junction.

Tubular sclerosis may obstruct the dentinal tubules causing their coronal ends to lose communication with the pulp. Therefore the tubules do not contain vital odontoblast processes and thus are 'dead tracts'. These tubules may contain gases, fluids, and degenerating cell remnants *in vivo*, but in ground sections they become readily filled with air and appear dark or opaque in transmitted light.

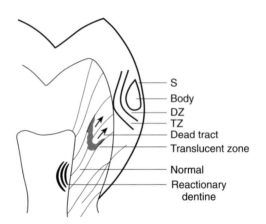

Fig. 3.6. Diagram of histological changes in enamel and dentine before cavitation of the enamel. S, Surfaces zone; Body, body of lesion; DZ, dark zone; TZ, translucent zone. (By courtesy of Professor N.W. Johnson.)

3.5.2 Histological appearance of the lesion after cavitation of the enamel

Once cavitation of the enamel occurs, bacteria have direct access to dentine and the tissue becomes infected. Figure 3.7 is a diagrammatic representa-

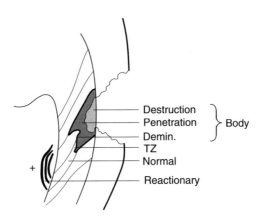

Fig. 3.7. Diagram of histological changes after cavitation. Note that demineralization of enamel precedes bacterial penetration. TZ, Translucent zone; DEMIN, demineralization. (By courtesy of Professor N.W. Johnson.)

tion of such a lesion. The three defence reactions of mild pulpal inflammation, reactionary dentine, and tubular sclerosis can be seen. The body of the lesion in dentine may now be divided into three structural components. At the advancing edge is an area of *demineralized dentine* which does not yet contain bacteria. Superficial to this is a *zone of penetration*, so called because the tubules have become penetrated by microorganisms. Superficial to this is a *zone of destruction* or necrosis where microbial action has completely destroyed the substance of the dentine.

The fact that demineralization precedes bacterial penetration is of great importance in operative dentistry, particularly in deep cavities, since a major objective is to remove the infected and necrotic tissue and then place a therapeutic lining material over the demineralized dentine. The object of this is to kill any bacteria remaining and encourage resolution of pulpal inflammation. The operative procedure is called *indirect pulp capping* and will be discussed further in Section 11.4.2.

Figures 3.8 and 3.9 show some histological appearances of carious dentine. In Fig. 3.8 a decalcified section of carious dentine stained with haematoxylin and eosin shows the deeply staining bacteria streaming down the dentinal tubules. Aggregations of bacteria and necrotic tissue coalesce to form *liquefaction foci* which appear to push the tubules apart. Destruction may also advance along the incremental lines of growth which are at right angles to the tubules to produce *transverse clefts* (Fig. 3.9).

In cross-section the bacteria can be seen in the tubules in Fig. 3.10 but in Fig. 3.11 destruction is more advanced and the bacteria are evident throughout the tissue.

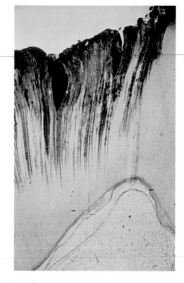

Fig. 3.8. Decalcified section of carious dentine showing dentinal tubules penetrated by deeply staining bacteria. In places the tubules appear to have been pushed apart by aggregations of bacteria called liquefaction foci. (By courtesy of Professor N.W. Johnson.)

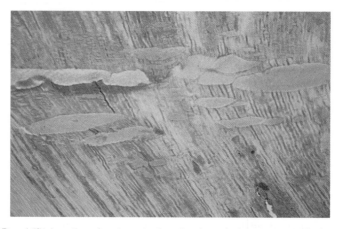

Fig. 3.9. Decalcified section of carious dentine showing tubules penetrated by bacteria. The tissue appears to have split at right angles to the tubules along the incremental lines of growth. These splits are called transverse clefts. (By courtesy of Professor N.W. Johnson.)

3.6 THE MICROBIOLOGY OF DENTINE CARIES

The first wave of bacteria infecting the dentine is primarily acidogenic. Since demineralization precedes bacterial penetration, the acid

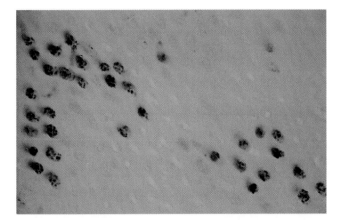

Fig. 3.10. A decalcified transverse section of carious dentine showing bacteria in the tubules. (By courtesy of Professor N.W. Johnson.)

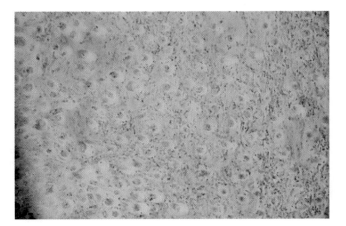

Fig. 3.11. A decalcified transverse section of carious dentine with bacteria evident throughout the tissue. (By courtesy of Professor N.W. Johnson.)

presumably diffuses ahead of the organisms. The pH of carious dentine can be low, and members of the dentine bacterial community tend to be more aciduric than those of supragingival plaque. When compared with the flora of supragingival plaque on intact enamel, infected dentine has higher proportions of gram-positive bacteria. Thus lactobacilli predominate with fewer mutans streptococci. The reasons for the ecological shift in the bacterial community could include the availability of the protein substrate and the low pH.

Within the zone of destruction there is a more mixed bacterial population, including organisms that can degrade proteins and peptides and degrade the dentine collagen. This collagen degradation is preceded by demineralization of the mineral fractions of dentine.

These ecological shifts within a carious cavity maybe of practical importance as well as academic interest. Once infected demineralized dentine is present within a cavity, removal of plaque from the surface of the tooth, by brushing or flossing, may no longer be sufficient to arrest the carious process. The infected demineralizing dentine must now be removed by operative treatment (see Section 11.2.1) and the cavity sealed with a restoration. Once this has been done removal of surface plaque may prevent recurrence of the carious process (see Section 11.2.4).

An interesting question that research workers have yet to answer is whether the carious process can be arrested by sealing over infected and demineralizing dentine. This would cut off the tissue from the oral environment but it is possible that the relevant microorganisms could survive and continue to destroy the dentine. Their source of nutrient would presumably be pulpal fluid. This possibility will be discussed again in Chapters 10 and 11.

3.7 ACTIVE AND ARRESTED LESIONS

The rate of progress of caries in dentine is highly variable and under suitable environmental conditions the carious process can be arrested and the lesion may even partly regress. Clinically, actively progressing lesions are soft and wet. Because of the speed of development of the lesion the defence reactions will not be well developed. Pain is easily evoked by hot, cold, and sweet stimuli. In contrast, arrested or slowly progressing lesions have a hard or leathery consistency. Histologically the defence reactions of reparative dentine and tubular sclerosis are marked. The body of the lesion in dentine accumulates organic matter and mineral from oral fluids, the most striking remineralization taking place on and within a surface exposed to the oral environment.

It is very important to realize that even caries of dentine does not automatically progress. Before the enamel surface is cavitated these lesions can be arrested by preventive treatment. It is a dentist's responsibility to explain to patients how they may arrest the disease in their mouths.

3.8 ROOT CARIES

Up to now this chapter has considered caries of dentine beneath enamel caries. However, in many mouths root surfaces become exposed to the oral environment by gingival recession and these surfaces are now susceptible to root caries and indeed are more vulnerable to mechanical and chemical destruction than enamel. Thus gingival recession is a prerequisite for exposure of a root surface, so it is hardly surprising that root caries is commonly seen in older people. It is associated with periodontal disease because this a major cause of gingival recession. However, this does not mean that all patients with exposed root surfaces will automatically get root caries since cariogenic plaque is the essential prerequisite.

Clinically both active (soft) and arrested or slowly progressing lesions (hard or leathery) may be seen. Active lesions are usually close to the gingival margin in the area of plaque stagnation. Note it is the consistency of the lesion, rather than its colour, which is the guide to its activity.

Early root surface lesions have been shown on microradiographs to be radiolucent zones (i.e. zones of demineralization) below a well mineralized surface layer which appears hypermineralized when compared with the neighbouring cementum. This hypermineralized surface zone covering early lesions is a consistent finding on exposed root surfaces but it is not present on non-exposed surfaces. This implies that mineral is likely to have precipitated from the saliva. Deep to the lesion there is frequently a hypermineralized area of tubular sclerosis and reparative dentine is seen at the pulpal surface of the dentine corresponding to the involved tubules.

Destruction of apatite crystals thus appears to take place below the surface before bacteria penetrate into the root cementum and dentine. In this respect enamel caries and root caries are similar. However, bacteria seem to penetrate into the tissue at an earlier stage in root caries than in coronal caries. Root lesions are very vulnerable to mechanical damage and probing should be almost totally avoided. It is also preferable to establish good plaque control but avoid root scaling until lesions have had the chance to arrest.

The recent dramatic decline in caries prevalence in children in many countries has resulted in an increased number of teeth being present in older individuals and for this reason root caries is of particular importance. The optimum management for root caries is again preventive treatment. Early diagnosis is important because active lesions may become arrested following improved plaque control with a fluoride toothpaste and care with diet. Root caries is particularly difficult to treat by operative means and this will be discussed further in Chapter 11.

REFERENCE

Thylstrup, A. and Fejerskov, O. (1994). *Textbook of clinical cariology*, (2nd edn), Ch. 6: Clinical and pathological features of dental caries. Munksgaard, Copenhagen.

4

Diagnosis and its relevance to management

4.1 INTRODUCTION

The diagnosis of dental caries is fundamental to the practice of dentistry. This chapter will discuss the problems of diagnosis, concentrating on the so-called 'early' carious lesion. The word 'early' has been written in inverted commas because such a lesion may have been present in the mouth for many years in an arrested state (see Chapter 1, p. 10 and Chapter 2, p. 28). An attempt will be made to answer four questions, namely:

1.   Why is the diagnosis of caries in its 'early' stages important?

2.   How can dental caries be diagnosed in its 'early' stages?
3.   How can the patient 'at risk' to active caries be diagnosed?
4.   What is the relevance of the diagnostic information to the management of the carious process?

4.2   WHY IS THE DIAGNOSIS OF CARIES IN ITS 'EARLY' STAGES IMPORTANT?

Early diagnosis of the carious lesion is important because the carious process can be modified by preventive treatment so that the lesion does not progress. If caries can be diagnosed at the stage of the white spot lesion the balance can be tipped in favour of arrest by modifying diet, improving plaque control, and sensible use of fluoride (see Fig. 1.14, p. 17).

So what is the 'point of no return' where we can no longer hope for arrest? At this point the restoration of damaged tissue by a filling material may be required. Perhaps the 'point of no return' is when a cavity is present, since a hole in the dental tissues is not expected to calcify up from the base and the cavity may trap plaque. Thus, one important question that the practitioner must answer is what will arrest and what must be restored? In addition, is it always possible to diagnose whether a cavity is present and of what relevance is this breach in the dental tissues?

4.3   HOW CAN DENTAL CARIES BE DIAGNOSED IN ITS 'EARLY' STAGES?

The diagnosis of caries in the surgery requires good lighting and dry, clean teeth. If heavy deposits of calculus or plaque are present, the mouth should be cleaned before attempting accurate diagnosis. Each quadrant of the mouth is isolated with cotton wool rolls to prevent saliva wetting the teeth once they have been dried. Thorough drying should be carried out with a gentle blast of air from the three-in-one syringe (see p. 20).

Sharp eyes can be used to look for the earliest signs of demineralization. Traditionally, sharp probes have also been used to detect the 'tacky' feel of early cavitation. However, this approach should NOT be used because a sharp probe can actually damage an incipient carious lesion (Fig. 4.1), and by carrying infected microorganisms into the lesion may facilitate spread of caries.

Good bitewing radiographs are also essential in diagnosis. In this technique the central beam of X-rays is positioned to pass at right angles to the long axis of the tooth, and tangentially through the contact area. The film is positioned in a film holder on the lingual side of the posterior teeth. The patient then closes the teeth together on the film holder. A beam-aiming

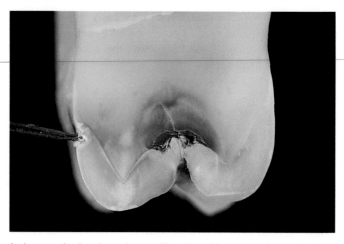

Fig. 4.1. A sharp probe has been jammed into the white spot lesion on the buccal aspect of this extracted molar. This picture shows the probe and the resulting damage. Figure 3.2 (p. 31) shows this lesion before probing.

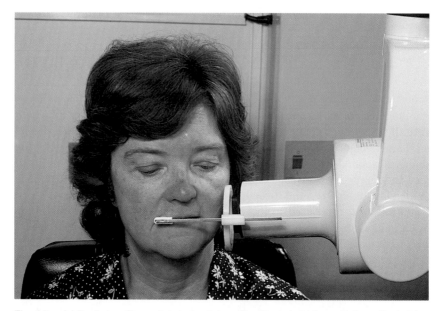

Fig. 4.2. A bitewing radiograph is being taken. The film is held lingually by a film holder and the patient closes together on a part of this holder. A beam aiming device helps the operator position the tube so that the beam is directed at right angles to the film.

device on the holder guides the position of the tube (Fig. 4.2). This directs the beam at right angles to the film and the contact areas of the teeth. The type of radiograph resulting can be seen in Fig. 4.3.

In order to answer the question of whether caries can be diagnosed in its 'early' stages and, if so, how this should be done, the individual sites where caries can occur must be considered separately. These are free smooth surfaces, pits and fissures, and approximal surfaces.

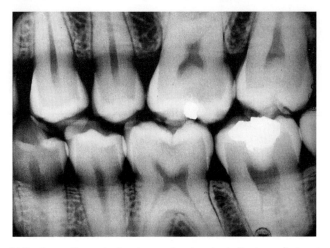

Fig. 4.3. A bitewing radiograph showing occlusal caries in the lower first molar. Clinically, there was no detectable cavity in this tooth although the enamel was discoloured.

4.3.1 Free smooth surfaces

Caries on free smooth *enamel* surfaces can be diagnosed with sharp eyes at the stage of the white or brown spot lesion (Fig. 1.4c, p. 6) before cavitation has occurred, provided the teeth are clean, dry, and well lit. Drying is very important because, as explained on p. 20 it gives the clinician an idea of the porosity of the lesion. Active lesions tend to be close to the gingival margin and may have a mat appearance indicative of surface loss of tissue (p. 6). Arrested lesions, on the other hand, may be left abandoned by the gingival margin and may have a shiny, lustrous surface. Sometimes these lesions are brown because the porosities have absorbed exogenous stain from the mouth (Fig. 2.2, p. 21).

Root surface caries, in its early stages, appears as one or more small, well defined, discoloured areas located in an area of plaque stagnation close to the gingival margin (Fig. 4.4). Lesions may vary in colour from yellowish or light brown, through midbrown to almost black. Active lesions are soft

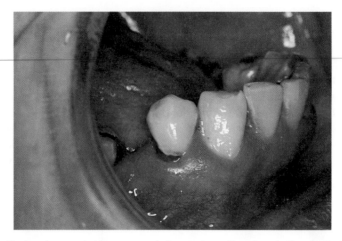

Fig. 4.4. Root surface caries in an area of plaque stagnation close to the gingival margin.

or leathery in consistency[1] and may cavitate. Arrested lesions are hard and are often located in a plaque-free area, coronal to the gingival margin (Fig. 4.5). Arrested lesions may be cavitated.

Although lesion consistency is important in diagnosing activity, great care should be taken when using a sharp instrument on these surfaces. A sharp probe could cause a small hole in which plaque will subsequently collect, possibly protected from the toothbrush bristle. It may be safer to test the consistency of the lesion by gentle use of an excavator. It should be

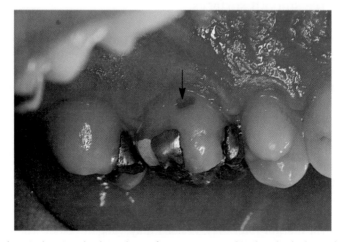

Fig. 4.5. Arrested root caries in a plaque-free area, coronal to the gingival margin.

noted that colour is not a good indicator of lesion activity. It seems likely that the colour of the lesion is due to exogenous staining from such items as tea, coffee, red wine, and chlorhexidine mouthwashes. Thus colour may reflect the use of these liquids rather than lesion activity.

Root surface lesions tend to spread laterally and coalesce with minor neighbouring lesions and may thus eventually encircle the tooth. Commonly, the lesions extend only 0.25–1 mm in depth. They do not always spread apically as the gingival margin recedes, but new lesions may develop later at the level of the new gingival margin. This may occur irrespective of an arrested lesion being located more coronally at the cement–enamel junction of the tooth.

4.3.2 Pits and fissures

While caries on free smooth surfaces is easy to see, caries in pits and fissures is difficult to diagnose at this early stage. The fissure which looks clinically caries-free may histologically show signs of early lesion formation. In addition, the fissure that is sticky to a sharp probe may not be carious histologically. The stickiness may indicate fissure shape or the pressure exerted rather than caries and, indeed, a sharp probe can actually damage an incipient carious lesion. For these reasons it is suggested that the probe must be reserved for removing any plaque from the fissure to allow sharp eyes to pick up discoloration, cavitation, and the grey appearance of enamel undermined by caries in the dentine beneath (Figs 4.6, 1.2, p. 5).

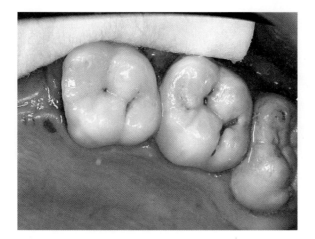

Fig. 4.6.   Occlusal caries in upper first and second molars.

In addition, bitewing radiographs are of great importance in the detection of occlusal caries, although by the time a lesion can be seen radiographically it is well into dentine (Fig. 4.3). Occlusal enamel may appear clinically caries-free[2] or slightly discoloured with no cavity to be seen or probed, but a bitewing radiograph may show caries in dentine.

Thus, to summarize, it is difficult to diagnose caries in pits and fissures reliably in its earliest stages and the anatomy of the area may favour spread of the lesion rather than lesion arrest. These facts are of considerable relevance in the management of caries in pits and fissures and will be discussed in Chapters 8 and 10.

In the future an electronic caries monitor (Fig. 4.7) may solve this diagnostic problem. Electrical resistance measurements[3] are a promising alternative method for diagnosis of occlusal caries. Intact enamel is a good insulator, but during the carious process, porosities form in the tissue which fill with water and ions from saliva. These moisture-filled porosities act as conductive pathways causing resistance values to fall. Research has shown that such measurements can detect demineralized lesions in occlusal enamel. Their value may be that they may be repeated on recall and comparative readings may indicate whether a lesion is progressing or not.

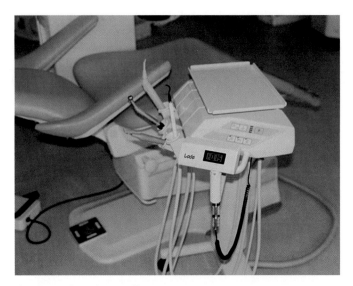

Fig. 4.7.   An electronic caries monitor.

4.3.3 Approximal surfaces

As with the fissure, it will be difficult to see the 'early' carious enamel lesion on an approximal surface. This is because the lesion forms just cervical to the contact area and vision is obscured by the adjacent tooth. The lesion is only discovered visually at a relatively late stage when it has already progressed into dentine and is seen as a pinkish grey area shining up through the marginal ridge (Fig. 1.3, p. 5). It must be emphasized again that the teeth should be isolated, clean, and dry to see this.

In contrast, an approximal lesion on the root surface may be diagnosed visually but gingival health is mandatory for such a diagnosis to be reliable. Thus, if the gingivae are red, swollen, and tending to bleed, caries diagnosis in these areas should be deferred until scaling, polishing, and improved oral hygiene have been instituted and the inflammation is resolved.

A sharp, curved probe (Briault) can be used gently to try to determine whether an approximal lesion is cavitated but if this instrument is used in a heavy-handed manner it can actually cause cavitation.

The bitewing radiograph is of paramount importance in the diagnosis of the approximal carious lesion (Fig. 4.8), although it should be remembered that the technique is relatively insensitive as it is not able to detect early subsurface demineralization. As shown diagrammatically in Fig. 4.9, the approximal enamel lesion appears as a dark triangular area in the enamel of the bitewing radiograph. The lesion may be in the outer enamel or be seen throughout the depth of the enamel. Larger lesions can be seen as a radiolucency in the enamel and outer half of the dentine or a radiolucency in the enamel reaching to the inner half of the dentine. The pulp is often exposed by the carious process in this latter instance.

Caries on the approximal root surface is also visible on a bitewing radiograph (Fig. 4.10) although this appearance is sometimes confused with

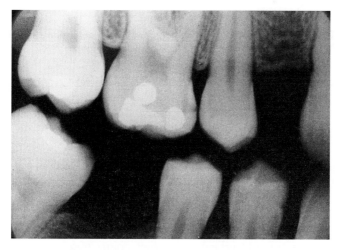

Fig. 4.8. A bitewing radiograph showing caries in enamel and dentine on the mesial aspect of the upper first molar. A lesion is also visible on the mesial aspect of the lower first premolar.

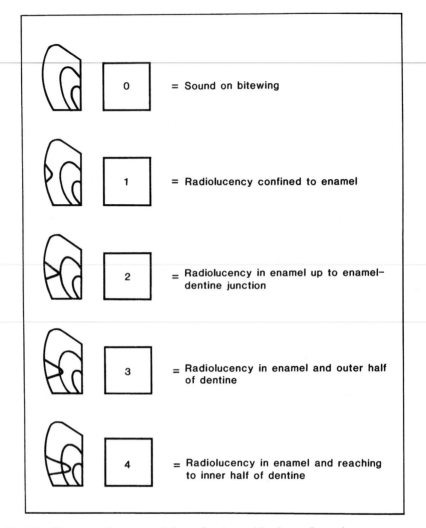

Fig. 4.9.   Diagrammatic representations of caries on bitewing radiographs.

the cervical radiolucency. The latter is a perfectly normal appearance caused by the absence of the dense enamel cap at the enamel–cement junction and absence of the interdental alveolar bone. Fortunately, root caries is visible clinically and a careful clinical re-examination will usually sort out any confusion.

It will be obvious that, to be of value, bitewing radiography must be carried out carefully. Overlapping contact points obscure what the clinician is trying to see and, unfortunately, slight differences in angulation of

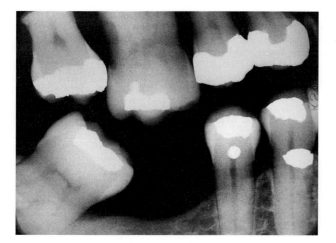

Fig. 4.10.   A bitewing radiograph showing root caries on the distal aspect of the first upper molar. This tooth has overerupted following loss of the lower first molar.

the film or X-ray beam will affect what is seen on the resultant radiograph. Thus radiographs should be as reproducible as possible, using film holders with beam-aiming devices (Fig. 4.2) and standardizing exposure time and dose. In addition films should be read dry, mounted, and under standardized lighting conditions.

Transmitted light can also be of considerable assistance in the diagnosis of approximal caries.[4] This technique consists of shining light through the contact point. A carious lesion has a lowered index of light transmission and therefore appears as a dark shadow that follows the outline of the decay through the dentine. The technique has been used for many years in the diagnosis of approximal lesions in anterior teeth. Light is reflected through the teeth using the dental mirror and carious lesions are readily seen in the mirror (Fig. 4.11).

In posterior teeth a stronger light source is required and fibreoptic lights, with the beam reduced to 0.5 mm in diameter, have been used (Fig. 4.12). It is important that the diameter of the light source is small so that glare and loss of surface detail are eliminated. The light should be used with the teeth dry. The technique is called fibreoptic transillumination (FOTI). It has particular advantages in patients with posterior crowding where bitewing radiographs will produce overlapping images and in pregnant women where unnecessary radiation should be avoided.

One further technique to assist with the diagnosis of approximal caries is the use of tooth separation.[5] This technique has been borrowed from the orthodontists who have used it for years to separate teeth before placing bands around them. A small round elastic is forced between the contact points using

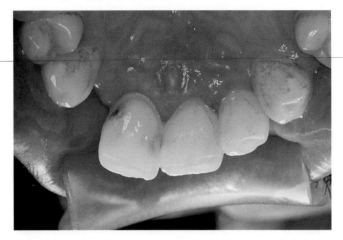

Fig. 4.11. A mirror view of the palatal aspect of the upper anterior teeth. Lesions are visible mesially and distally on the upper right central incisor.

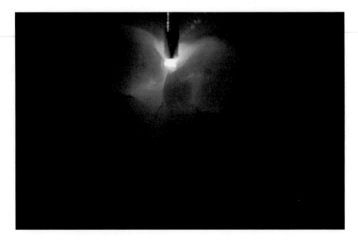

Fig. 4.12. Use of a fibreoptic light in the diagnosis of approximal caries. (By courtesy of Dr C. Pine.)

a special pair of applicating forceps (Fig. 4.13a). After a few days the teeth are separated (Fig. 4.13b). Sometimes the dentist can now see the approximal area by direct vision and feel it, *very gently*, with a probe to detect whether a cavity is present. A better way of detecting a cavity is to inject a little elastomer impression material between the teeth (Fig. 4.13c). After a few minutes the set material can be removed with a probe and the impression examined to see whether there in a cavity (Fig. 4.13d).

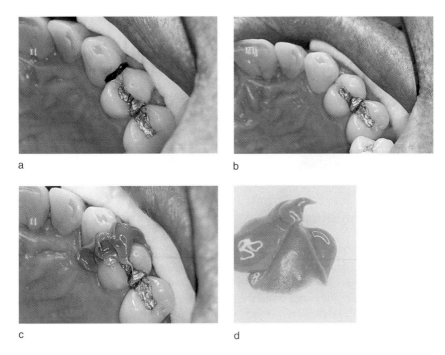

Fig. 4.13. (a) Orthodontic separator in place between the canine and first premolar. The dentist is unsure whether a restoration is required on the distal surface of the canine. (b) Separation achieved 48 hours later. Note it is not possible to see the distal surface of the canine clearly. (c) Taking an elastomer impression of the contact area. (d) Elastomer impression of the contact area showing no cavitation on the distal aspect of the canine; a restoration is not needed.

4.4 HOW CAN THE PATIENT 'AT RISK' TO ACTIVE CARIES BE DIAGNOSED?

It has already been stressed that caries should not be regarded purely as a process of demineralization but as an alternating process of destruction, arrest, and partial repair. If the process can be diagnosed early the dentist can help the patient institute preventive measures to tip the balance in favour of arrest. However, diagnosis implies more than just recording the number of cavities, their location, and appearance. The dentist needs to know whether the patient is likely to develop new cavities and/or whether existing cavities are likely to progress.

This concept may be illustrated by two examples. Imagine examining a five-year-old child for the first time. The dentition appears clinically caries-free. Does this patient need advice on prevention of disease or merely praise for doing so well? Now consider a 60-year-old patient, again seen for the first time; the mouth is fairly heavily restored and there is evidence of root caries on some teeth. Are these lesions likely to progress or have they already arrested? The dentist needs to know this before deciding how best to manage the patient. Thus the prudent practitioner will make a caries risk assessment on all patients when they initially present, recording risk as high, low, or intermediate. This assessment should be updated at each recall visit since the patient's circumstances may change. Caries risk assessment is a complex topic. Figure 4.14 lists some of the many factors to be considered so that through a careful history, clinical examination and special tests, this risk assessment may be made.

4.4.1 Social history

Dental caries is now principally a problem for the socially deprived. Social factors will be assessed, often subconsciously, as the patient enters the room. Dress, demeanour, and ethnic background will be apparent for subjective appraisal, although care must be taken not to jump to unwarranted and inaccurate conclusions. Questions on employment, work pattern such as shift work, attendance pattern of other family members, elicit valuable information. During history-taking the patient's dental aspirations become apparent and relevant treatment planning will encompass these aspirations. Life changes such as a move from home to boarding school or university, a change from employment to unemployment, retirement, and bereavement may all affect eating patterns and therefore caries status.

4.4.2 Medical history

Medical history is always important in dental practice and some illnesses specifically predispose to a high risk of dental caries. The most important of these are medical problems causing dry mouth (xerostomia) such as radiotherapy in the region of the salivary glands, Sjögren's syndrome (see Chapter 5, pp. 69), and long term use of some medications such as tranquillizers, antihypertensives, and diuretics. Frequent medication may of itself pose a risk if the medication is sugar-based.

4.4.3 Dietary habits

Dietary habits, and the patient's attitudes to them, are of importance. A diet analysis may be a useful piece in the information jigsaw and the various techniques of diet analysis will be discussed in detail in Chapter 6.

CARIES RISK ASSESSMENT

HIGH RISK	LOW RISK
SOCIAL HISTORY	
Socially deprived	Middle class
High caries in siblings	Low caries in siblings
Low knowledge of dental disease	Dentally aware
Irregular attender	Regular attender
Ready availability snacks	Work does not allow regular snacks
Low dental aspirations	High dental aspirations
MEDICAL HISTORY	
Medically compromised	No medical problem
Handicapped	No physical problem
Xerostomia	Normal salivary flow
Long term cariogenic medicine	No long term medication
DIETARY HABITS	
Frequent sugar intake	Infrequent sugar intake
USE OF FLUORIDE	
Drinking water not fluoridated	Drinking water fluoridated
No fluoride supplements	Fluoride supplements used
No fluoride toothpaste	Fluoride toothpaste used
PLAQUE CONTROL	
Infrequent, ineffective cleaning	Frequent, effective cleaning
Poor manual control	Good manual control
SALIVA	
Low flow rate	Normal flow rate
Low buffering capacity	High buffering capacity
High *S.mutans* and lactobacillus counts	Low *S.mutans* and lactobacillus counts
CLINICAL EVIDENCE	
New lesions	No new lesions
Premature extractions	Nil extractions for caries
Anterior caries or restorations	Sound anterior teeth
Multiple restorations	No or few restorations
History repeated restorations	Restorations inserted years ago
No fissure sealants	Fissure sealed
Multiband orthodontics	No appliance
Partial dentures	

Fig. 4.14.   Caries risk assessment.

4.4.4 Use of fluoride

History of fluoride use is also of importance since the fluoride ion delays lesion progression. Practitioners will know the fluoride content of the local water supply. However, only about 10 per cent of the population of the United Kingdom have access to fluoridated water so that the most common fluoride supplement is fluoride toothpaste. Although fluoride toothpaste is used by most people, it is always wise to check. It is surprising how often a patient with multiple carious lesions has selected a particular brand of toothpaste, manufactured for sensitive teeth, which does not contain fluoride.

4.4.5 Plaque control

Since bacterial plaque is responsible for the carious process, poor oral hygiene is a caries risk. This will be discussed in detail in Chapter 8.

4.4.6 Saliva

Saliva is a protective fluid as far as the mouth is concerned. A low secretion rate leads to reduced elimination of microorganisms and food remnants, impaired neutralization of acids and a reduced ability to repair the early enamel lesion. A low salivary secretion rate is generally accompanied by a low buffer capacity and an increased number of mutans streptococci and lactobacilli. Thus increased caries activity is seen in persons with a reduced salivary secretion rate. This will be discussed in more detail in Chapter 5.

Unstimulated salivary secretion rate can be determined by the patient sitting quietly in the dental chair, without chewing or swallowing but spitting into a disposable cup.

Stimulated salivary secretion rate can be determined in the following way. The patient is asked to swallow any saliva present in the mouth and then to chew on a piece of folded-over paraffin film. Saliva formed over the next five minutes is expectorated into a disposable cup. The volume of saliva secreted is measured by aspirating the saliva into a disposable, plastic, graduated syringe (Fig. 4.15). The secretion rate is then expressed in millilitres per minute. When the secretion rate is very low the saliva collected may also be frothy and difficult to measure. In such cases the addition of a measured amount of water will eliminate the froth and so facilitate measurement.

Normal unstimulated secretion rate in adults	0.3–0.5 ml/min
Normal stimulated secretion rate in adults	1–2 ml/min

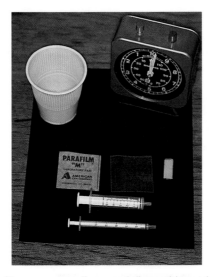

Fig. 4.15. Paraffin film, paper cup, timer, and disposable graduated syringes (1 and 5 ml) for measurement of salivary flow.

Low stimulated secretion rate in adults	<0.7 ml/min
Severely dry mouth	<0.1 ml/min.

Some of the paraffin-stimulated saliva can now be used to give an indication of the buffering capacity provided the saliva was not diluted. Since the buffering capacity of saliva generally increases after eating, it is preferable to collect samples about two hours after a meal. Special kits are commercially available (Ivoclar Vivadent Ltd) which are convenient for chairside use. A simple litmus-type test measures buffering capacity. The litmus paper is dipped in the patient's saliva and the colour is compared with the manufacturer's chart to read off the patient's buffering capacity (Fig. 4.16).

Normal buffering capacity	final pH 5–7
Low buffering capacity	final pH 4.

If salivary examination shows low values for secretion rate and buffering capacity, tests should be repeated to determine whether the values are occasional or constant. If they are constant, the causative factor has to be determined (Chapter 5).

Some microorganisms are more important than others in the pathogenesis of dental caries. There is now some evidence that individuals with a low level of mutans streptococci may be at low risk to dental caries. In addition, there is some evidence that a high level of lactobacilli is associ-

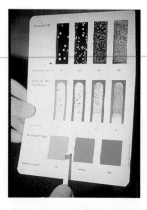

Fig. 4.16. A proprietary kit used to estimate buffering capacity. The litmus paper is dipped in the patient's saliva and the colour is compared with the manufacturer's chart to read off the patient's buffering capacity. (Reproduced by courtesy of Ivoclar Vivadent Ltd.)

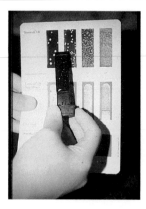

Fig. 4.17. A proprietary kit used to estimate a lactobacillus count. The dip slide is covered with the patient's saliva and incubated. It is then compared with the manufacturer's chart to estimate the lactobacillus count. (Reproduced by courtesy of Ivoclar Vivadent Ltd.)

ated with a cariogenic diet. High levels of this organism are also associated with multiple open cavities, and such cavities should be excavated and temporarily dressed (Chapter 11) before determining the level of lactobacillus infection. Commercially available kits are available to assess both mutans streptococci and lactobacilli (Ivoclar Vivadent Ltd). The authors reserve bacterial counts for the management of xerostomic patients who are a very high caries risk.

The commercial kit used to assess the lactobacillus count consists of a slide inoculated with a special medium to allow lactobacilli to grow.

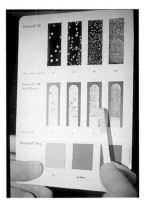

Fig. 4.18. A proprietary kit used to estimate a *Streptococcus mutans* count. The spatula is rotated on the patient's tongue and incubated in a special culture medium. It is then compared with the manufacturer's chart to estimate the *Streptococcus mutans* count. (Reproduced by courtesy of Ivoclar Vivadent Ltd.)

Paraffin-stimulated saliva is collected from the patient and poured over the slide which is incubated, and any lactobacilli in the saliva multiply to form colonies on the slide. The number of colonies can then be estimated by reference to the manufacturer's chart (Fig. 4.17). A similar system is available for estimation of *Streptococcus mutans*, although in this case saliva is collected by rotating a special slide on the patient's tongue (Fig. 4.18).

4.4.7 Clinical evidence

Clinical evidence is the most useful indicator of caries risk.[6] A history of repeated restoration and re-restoration, together with multiple new lesions on clinical and/or radiographic examination, is an obvious caries risk. If the mucosa is dry and dull a reduced salivary flow may be suspected. The presence of large amounts of plaque and the state of the periodontium will also give us some clues. Root surfaces exposed as a result of periodontal disease may be susceptible to caries. Stagnation areas, such as erupting occlusal surfaces, unsealed deep fissures, multiband orthodontic appliances, partial dentures, and poor restorative dentistry, encourage plaque accumulation and increase caries risk.

It is important when caries is recorded that its localization and appearance is noted as well as its prevalence. For example, if caries is present in the lower anterior teeth, the caries risk is greater than if only the fissures of posterior teeth are involved. Hard lesions would not concern the dentist as much as soft lesions. Recurrent caries around existing restorations should also sound warning bells.

4.4.8 Assessment of findings

For assessment of the actual caries risk, information from the case history and the clinical and radiographic examination, the dietary history, and the salivary tests all have to be considered. No single negative factor should be taken to imply a high caries risk. A plaque-covered surface will not inevitably develop a cavity. Although sugar consumption and the number of mutans streptococci are closely associated with caries, there are many people with high counts who do not develop caries. Similarly, some people can eat sugar frequently but be caries-free. The carious process is caused by several factors and must be treated as such.

4.5 THE RELEVANCE OF THE DIAGNOSTIC INFORMATION TO THE MANAGEMENT OF THE CARIOUS PROCESS

It is important to remember that clinical and radiographic diagnoses may be inaccurate and inconsistent. No one can be sure of recording the same caries diagnosis on different occasions on one patient, and to prove the point the student might like to collect a number of bitewing radiographs, note their findings and then repeat the exercise a week later. Students will find they are not always consistent with themselves, let alone a colleague. However, they should not feel too despondent about this since the trained epidemiologist is only 70–80 per cent reliable!

When carious lesions are diagnosed the clinician must decide how the process should be treated. Currently there are two possible approaches:

1. To use preventive measures to attempt to arrest the process.
2. Surgically to remove and replace the damaged tissues and prevent recurrence.

These two approaches will now be considered in the light of the diagnostic information available.

4.5.1 Free smooth surfaces

Caries on free smooth surfaces can be diagnosed at the stage of the white spot lesion, that is before cavitation occurs. However, on the first occasion dentist and patient meet, it may not be obvious whether such a lesion represents active decay or a chronic static lesion which has been present for many years. Thus although it is easy to diagnose, it may not be easy to interpret. The wise practitioner will probably discuss the problem with the patient and carry out diet analysis. Preventive measures such as dietary advice (Chapter 6), use of fluoride (Chapter 7), and improved plaque control (Chapter 8) can then be instituted and the lesion reassessed in six months.

4.5.2 Pits and fissures

Since caries in pits and fissures is difficult to diagnose in its earliest stage and since fissures are particularly susceptible sites, the dentist may decide to fissure-seal susceptible teeth as soon after eruption as possible. Fissure sealants are materials which cover and protect the fissure and are discussed in detail in Chapter 10.

The occlusal lesion which shows on a bitewing radiograph (Fig. 4.3) should be restored (Chapter 11). A small occlusal restoration, carefully executed, is preferable to the risk of waiting until an exposure necessitates root canal therapy. The anatomy of the fissure and the consequent shape of the carious lesion often results in gross undermining of enamel by the carious process.

4.5.3 Approximal surfaces

In epidemiological studies, ranking systems are used which divide enamel and dentine into inner and outer halves so that a more sensitive indication of lesion depth is possible. One such system is illustrated in Fig. 4.9 and will be used to discuss the clinical problem of when to restore. Teeth that are sound on radiograph (0) will be left alone, although it must still be remembered that early white spots may still be present, the radiographic technique being less sensitive than the naked eye.

A lesion limited to the enamel on bitewing radiograph should be treated preventively. Histologically these lesions are probably in dentine but are unlikely to be cavitated: thus preventive measures should arrest the lesion. Time is on the patient's side unless the caries risk is very high. Research has shown that progression of a lesion through enamel, if it occurs, can be very slow, taking two to six years before it is evident in dentine radiographically.[7]

Whether to cut or attempt to arrest the lesion which on radiograph is through enamel and just into dentine is a more difficult clinical decision. Some of these lesions will be cavitated but others will not[8] and this break in the enamel surface cannot be diagnosed from the radiographic appearance. This is the lesion where tooth separation and an impression (Fig. 4.13a–d) may be justified. Knowing whether there is a cavity is important because cavities will not 'fill up from the bottom' and logic suggests that the lesion may not arrest unless the plaque in the cavity can be removed. A cavity will be a plaque trap if it is not accessible to a toothbrush and dental floss or tape will not enter the hole. Usually a decision is made on the radiographic appearance alone. In young patients or high- and medium-risk patients the authors would treat operatively. In a low-risk patient (like *you*, our dental reader!) we would suggest preventive treatment, showing you the radiographic picture and suggesting it should be repeated in six months.

Teeth that are very carious on radiograph should be restored and measures instituted to prevent recurrence. A periapical radiograph should be taken to check whether the carious process has resulted in pulp necrosis and an area of chronic periapical infection. If this is the case, root canal treatment will be required if the tooth is to be saved.

4.5.4 Root caries

Early diagnosis of root caries is of particular clinical importance because advanced disease is virtually impossible to treat by operative means. Lesions coalesce to encircle the neck of the tooth and eventually the crown may break off.

Previous root surface caries experience and salivary flow rate have been shown to be good predictors of the risk of root caries. A combination of meticulous plaque control, dietary control, and use of topical fluoride (as a varnish and/mouthwash) should be used to prevent the development of new lesions.

Using such an approach, it may be possible to reharden even rather extensive root caries. In this connection it should be remembered that although the lesions may be extensive, they are usually shallow. As the lesions become arrested there may also be slight cavitation as soft material is brushed away. Vigorous probing of active root carious lesions should be avoided so as not to impair the surface of the tooth.

Root caries should be treated operatively to aid plaque control, to improve appearance, and where lesions are deep to protect the pulp.

4.5.5 Deciduous teeth

The majority of what has been written about the diagnosis and management of caries in the permanent dentition is applicable to the deciduous dentition. For instance, it is just as important to use bitewing radiographs for diagnosis of caries in deciduous teeth as in permanent teeth. However, there are some obvious differences which are worth stressing:

1. Deciduous teeth are smaller than permanent teeth; the pulps are relatively large in proportion to the enamel and dentine.
2. For this reason the disease may pass through enamel and dentine and affect the pulp more rapidly than in the permanent dentition.
3. The caries-susceptible child should thus be examined frequently and operative intervention may be advisable earlier than in the permanent dentition.
4. Since deciduous teeth are small, operative dentistry may be difficult if lesions are too large. For this reason many paediatric dentists would advise operative treatment of approximal lesions which have reached the enamel–dentine junction.
5. Deciduous teeth do not usually develop root caries unless they are retained into adult life when their roots may become exposed and therefore vulnerable.

REFERENCES

1. Hellyer, P.H., Beighton, D., Heath, M.R., and Lynch, E.J.R. (1990). Root caries in older people attending a general dental practice in East Sussex. *Br. Dent. J.*, **169**, 201–6.
2. Weerheijm, K.L., Groen, H.J., Bast, A.J.J., Kieft, J.A., Eijkman, M.A.J., and van Amerongen, W.E. (1992). Clinically undetected occlusal dentine caries: a radiographic comparison. *Caries Res.*, **26**, 305–9.
3. Ricketts, D.N.J., Kidd, E.A.M., and Wilson, R.F. (1995). A re-evaluation of electrical resistance measurements for the diagnosis of occlusal caries. *Br. Dent. J.*, **178**, 11–17.
4. Mitropoulos, C.M. (1985). A comparison of fibreoptic transillumination with bitewing radiographs. *Br. Dent. J.*, **159**, 21–3.
5. Pitts, N.B. and Longbottom, C. (1987). Temporary tooth separation with special reference to the diagnosis and preventive management of equivocal approximal carious lesions. *Quintessence Int.*, **18**, 563–73.
6. Pienihakkinen, K. (1987). Caries prediction through combined use of incipient carious lesions, salivary buffering capacity, lactobacilli and yeasts in Finland. *Community Dent. Oral Epidemiol.*, **15**, 325–8.
7. Pitts, N.B. (1983). Monitoring of caries progression in permanent and primary approximal enamel by bitewing radiography. A review. *Community Dent. Oral Epidemiol.*, **11**, 228–35.
8. Seddon, R.P. (1989). The detection of cavitation in carious approximal surfaces *in vivo* by tooth separation, impression and scanning electron microscopy. *J. Dent.*, **17**, 117–20.

5

Saliva and caries

5.1 INTRODUCTION

Saliva is a complex oral fluid consisting of a mixture of secretions from the major salivary glands and the minor glands of the oral mucosa. Ninety per cent of saliva is produced by the three pairs of major glands: parotid, submandibular, and sublingual. The rest of the saliva is produced by thousands of minor salivary glands distributed throughout the mouth and throat. Most of the saliva is produced at mealtimes as a response to stimulation due to tasting and chewing (stimulated saliva). For the rest of the day, although salivary flow is low, it is extremely important. In healthy individuals under resting conditions, without the stimulation associated with chewing, there is a constant slow flow of saliva which moistens and helps to protect the teeth, tongue, and mucous membranes of the mouth and oropharynx (resting saliva). The flow rate peaks during the afternoon and virtually stops during sleep. This has important clinical implications for the timing of oral hygiene. Since plaque and food debris and a greatly reduced salivary flow provide ideal conditions for dental caries, the most important time of day to clean teeth is at night before going to sleep.

The normal resting or *unstimulated* secretion rate in adults is between 0.3 and 0.5 ml per minute. The normal *stimulated* secretion rate in adults is 1-2 ml per minute. However, the rates may be reduced to less than 0.1 ml per minute or may not be measurable in individuals with severe salivary gland malfunction. The terms *xerostomia* (Greek: xeros = dry; stoma = mouth) and *dry mouth* are used to describe this condition. In less severe cases of hyposalivation the stimulated secretion rate is between 0.7 and 0.1 ml per minute.

The composition and viscosity of saliva depends on the relative contributions from the various salivary glands. Although they are similar in structure, the viscosity of the secretions they produce varies. Parotid secretions are watery and clear while the minor glands in the mouth and throat produce secretions that are 9 times more viscous and 45 times more ropey. The secretions produced by the submandibular and sublingual glands are respectively two and three times more viscous than parotid saliva. Under normal conditions the parotid glands produce 50 per cent of the stimulated saliva and 20 per cent of the resting saliva. Most of the resting saliva is produced by the submandibular (65 per cent), sublingual (7–8 per cent) and minor salivary glands (7–8 per cent). Resting saliva is therefore more viscous than stimulated saliva. It becomes even more viscous and ropey when only the minor glands contribute. Such saliva is uncomfortable for the patient because it makes swallowing difficult.

5.2 SALIVA AND DENTAL HEALTH[1,2]

5.2.1 Functions of saliva

Although saliva aids swallowing and digestion, and is required for optimal function of the taste buds, its most important role is to maintain the integrity of the teeth, tongue, and mucous membranes of the oral and oropharyngeal regions. Its protective action is manifested in several ways:

1. It forms a protective mucoid coating on the mucous membrane which acts as a barrier to irritants and prevents desiccation.
2. Its flow helps to clear the mouth of food and cellular and bacterial debris and consequently retards plaque formation.
3. It is capable of regulating the pH of the oral cavity by virtue of its bicarbonate content as well as its phosphate and amphoteric protein constituents. An increase in secretion rate usually results in an increase in pH and buffering capacity. The mucous membrane is thus protected

from acid in food or vomit. In addition the fall in plaque pH, as a result of the action of acidogenic organisms, is minimized.

4. It helps to maintain the integrity of teeth in several ways because of its calcium and phosphate content. It provides minerals which are taken up by the incompletely formed enamel surface soon after eruption (post-eruptive maturation). Tooth dissolution is prevented or retarded and remineralization is enhanced by the presence of a copious salivary flow. The film of glycoprotein formed on the tooth surface by saliva (the acquired pellicle) may also protect the tooth by reducing wear due to erosion and abrasion.

5. Saliva is capable of considerable antibacterial and antiviral activity by virtue of its content of specific antibodies (secretory IgA) as well as lysozyme, lactoferrin, and lactoperoxidase.

5.2.2 Causes of reduced salivary flow

There are numerous systemic conditions (listed in Table 5.1) which can alter the salivary flow rate. However, the most serious causes of malfunction of the salivary glands are radiotherapy in the region of these glands, drugs, and disease.

Radiotherapy

The exposure of the salivary glands to radiation during radiotherapy for neoplasms in the head and neck region usually results in a severe reduction in salivary flow (less than 0.1 ml/min.). When the parotid glands are

Table 5.1 Systemic causes of 'dry mouth'

Drugs
Psychological factors
Sjögren's syndrome
Hormonal changes (pregnancy, post-menopause)
Diabetes mellitus
Dehydration
Neurological diseases
Pancreatic disturbances
Liver disturbances
Nutritional deficiencies (anorexia nervosa, malnutrition)
Systemic lupus erythematosis
Immunodeficiency disease (AIDS)
Duct calculi
Smoking
?Ageing

involved, there is also a considerable increase in its total protein content resulting in a thick, viscous secretion which makes the condition even more uncomfortable. The time taken for salivary flow rate to return towards normal values varies and depends on the individual as well as the dose to which the glands have been exposed. Thus, in some patients, there is a considerable improvement after three months while in others xerostomia may be permanent as a result of atrophy of the glands induced by the radiation.

Drugs

A large number of therapeutic drugs affect salivary flow rate as well as its composition. Listed in Table 5.2 are the groups of drugs which result in decreased flow. Consequently, if any of them are used for more than a few weeks, steps must be taken to protect the teeth from caries. In addition, chemotherapy with cytotoxic drugs used in the management of some malignancies may also cause acute onset of dry mouth.

Table 5.2 Medications which retard salivary flow

Antidepressants	Diuretics
Antipsychotic drugs	Anti-Parkinsonian drugs
Tranquillizers	Appetite suppressants
Hypnotics	Antinauseants
Antihistamines	Antiemetics
Anticholinergics	Muscle relaxants
Antihypertensives	Expectorants

Disease

Acute and chronic inflammation of the salivary glands (sialadenitis), benign or malignant tumours as well as Sjögren's syndrome, may all lead to xerostomia depriving the individual of the protective action of saliva. Sjögren's syndrome is an autoimmune connective tissue disorder. It affects principally the salivary and lacrymal glands which become damaged by lymphocytic infiltrates and therefore produce less secretion. Fifteen to thirty per cent of patients with rheumatoid arthritis also have Sjögren's syndrome. For this reason the possibility of a dry mouth should be considered in patients with rheumatoid arthritis.

Age

It is generally assumed that a reduction in salivary flow is the inevitable result of ageing. However, recent studies show that at least for the parotid gland flow, there is no diminution of stimulated fluid output with increasing age in healthy subjects not on therapeutic drugs. On the other hand, there is some evidence that atrophic changes can occur in submandibular glands with age, which could result in reduced flow and small changes in composition of the saliva. It would seem, therefore, that any small decrease in salivary flow as a result of ageing is very slight compared with reductions in flow due to disease and the use of drugs in this group of individuals.

5.2.3 General consequences of reduced salivary flow

The useful role of saliva is not usually appreciated until there is a shortage. The contribution that saliva makes to oral health is therefore best demonstrated by examining the consequences of xerostomia. The oral mucosa, without the lubricating and protective action of saliva, is more prone to traumatic ulceration and infection. Mucositis presents as tenderness, pain, or a burning sensation and is exacerbated by spicy foods, fruits, alcoholic and carbonated beverages, hot drinks, and tobacco. Taste sensation is altered, and chewing and swallowing present difficulties, particularly if the food is bulky or dry. When salivary flow is diminished foods requiring a great deal of chewing are not well tolerated. This makes matters worse because chewing itself helps to stimulate salivary flow, provided there is some glandular activity left. Speaking may become difficult because of lack of lubrication. These individuals also suffer from extreme sensitivity of teeth to heat and cold, especially if any dentine is exposed. Edentulous patients may have problems tolerating dentures, probably because of reduction in surface tension between the dry mucosa and the fitting surface of the denture.

There is an increase in dental plaque accumulation which makes gingivitis more likely. However, there is no evidence that periodontitis, which involves loss of bone support, is affected. There is also modification of the plaque flora in favour of *Candida*, mutans streptococci and lactobaccilli. Consequently, in patients with dry mouths, candidal infections are frequent and rampant caries is common if no preventive measures are taken. 'Radiation caries' will be discussed in detail later (see Section 5.4.2).

5.3 CLINICAL MANAGEMENT OF 'DRY MOUTH'

5.3.1 Assessment

Drug history

As a first step, the patient's drug history should the checked since all the medications listed in Table 5.2 can adversely affect salivary flow and consequently aggravate the problem. New formulations are often prescribed so it is always wise to check with the National Formulary for any side effects. If any of these drugs are being taken for long periods it may be advisable for a dentist to contact the patient's medical practitioner to see whether the drug regime could be modified.

It is also relevant to check whether the patient is using a mouthwash since some of them contain up to 27 per cent alcohol and can therefore cause further discomfort. If the alcohol content of a mouthwash is not stated on the bottle the dentist should contact the manufacturer for this information.

Salivary flow measurements

It is important to standardize the time of day at which saliva is collected since the flow rate peaks during the afternoon. The patient should not eat or drink (except water) for at least one hour before collection. Measurement of unstimulated and stimulated flow rates and buffer capacity should be determined as described in Section 4.4.6. This will help to assess the extent of the problem by providing a quantitative assessment of an individual's salivary gland function and can be used to monitor the course of the disease. A simple comparison of the stimulated and unstimulated rate will indicate if the glands are capable of being stimulated.

5.3.2 Salivary stimulants

Having established the extent of impairment, the next step is to try to increase salivary flow.

Salivary stimulants will only be helpful when there is some glandular activity present. The following agents have been used:

1. Chewing gum or sucking acidic sweets may increase salivary flow. However, if a patient is dentate anything acidic is contraindicated. Some fruit drops flavoured with artificial sweeteners normally marketed for diabetics are very acidic and may dissolve enamel and dentine. However, chewing a sugar-free gum, particularly one containing xylitol will incease salivary flow safely (see p. 96).
2. 'Salivix' is a proprietary lozenge containing malic acid, gum arabic, calcium lactate, sodium phosphate, lycasin, and sorbitol. The manufacturers claim that it stimulates salivary flow and that, because of the calcium lactate buffer present, it does not demineralize enamel in spite of a pH of 4.0. However, since it has not been tested on dentine, more work is required before it can be recommended for dentate patients.
3. The systemic use of drugs such as pilocarpine hydrochloride has proved successful in stimulating saliva in some cases. However, it does not restore lost glandular function and should be used with caution because of poten-

tial unpleasant side effects. Pilocarpine reproduces the effects of wide-spread stimulation of the parasympathetic nervous system. Conseqently, as well as stimulating saliva and tear production it can cause sweating, flushing, nausea, and diarrhoea. It can also slow the pulse rate, producing a fall in blood pressure and cause reflex narrowing of airways. It is therefore contraindicated in patients with cardiac or chest problems.

The recommended dose is four drops of a 1 per cent ophthalmic solution, taken orally, four times a day. However, the dose can be adjusted according to response and side effects and most patients only use it before bed, before a speaking engagement or before going out for a meal. The onset of action is usually 10–30 minutes and the effect lasts between one and four hours.

5.3.3 Saliva substitutes

In the past, individuals with dry mouth have had to rely on frequent moistening with water or liquids such as liquid paraffin or glycerine. Several saliva substitutes are now available to make the patient feel more comfortable and ideally to supply calcium, phosphate, and fluoride ions to aid remineralization. Saliva substitutes have been produced in the form of a spray or lozenge.

Sprays

The following preparations are commercially available in the UK: Luborant (Antigen International Ltd), Saliva Orthana (Nycomed, UK Ltd) and Glandosane (Dylade Company Ltd). They all contain calcium, phosphate, sodium, magnesium, and potassium ions. However, while Luborant and Glandosane contain carboxymethyl cellulose to provide viscosity, Saliva Orthana contains mucin prepared from the gastric mucosa of the pig. The other important difference between them is that while Luborant and Saliva Orthana both contain fluoride, have a pH between 6 and 7 and have been shown to have a significant remineralizing capacity *in vitro*, Glandosane does not contain fluoride and has a somewhat lower pH at 5.1. Glandosane should, therefore, be used only for edentulous patients. The sprays should be directed towards the inside of the cheeks and not down the throat.

Lozenges

Lozenges are only helpful if there is enough saliva present to dissolve them. Saliva Orthana is also available in the form of a lozenge. It does not contain fluoride but is quite palatable.

Salad oil

Some patients get relief by spreading salad oil around the mouth last thing at night.

Viscous or ropey saliva

When saliva is present but is ropey, rinsing or gargling with a mouthwash made up by mixing half a teaspoonful of salt and one teaspoonful of baking powder with one litre of warm water will break up the mucous in the mouth and throat.

Unfortunately, there has been no controlled study to date comparing the acceptability and effectiveness of these preparations so that no particular one can be recommended. Indeed, none of these agents is ideal and some patients still resort to filling spray bottles with water to be used at frequent intervals. However, it is obvious that any preparation with a low pH should never be used for dentate patients. Ideally, the saliva substitute should contain fluoride and be supplemented by a daily fluoride mouthwash (see p. 115).

5.4 SALIVA AND CARIES

5.4.1 Anti-cariogenic action of saliva

Theoretically saliva can influence the carious process in several ways:

1. The flow of saliva can reduce plaque accummulation on the tooth surface and also increase the rate of carbohydrate clearance from the oral cavity.
2. The diffusion into plaque of salivary components such as calcium, phosphate, hydroxyl, and fluoride ions can reduce the solubility of enamel and promote remineralization of early carious lesions.
3. The carbonic acid–bicarbonate buffering system, as well as ammonia and urea constituents of the saliva, can buffer and neutralize the pH fall which occurs when plaque bacteria metabolize sugar. The pH and buffering capacity of saliva is related to its secretion rate. The pH of patotid saliva increases from about 5.5 for unstimulated saliva to about 7.4 when the flow rate is high. The respective pH values for submandibular saliva are 6.4 and 7.1. An increase in the secretion rate of saliva also results in a greater buffering capacity. In both cases this is due to the increase in sodium and bicarbonate concentrations.
4. Several non-immunological components of saliva such as lysozyme, lactoperoxidase, and lactoferrin have a direct antibacterial action on

plaque microflora or may affect their metabolism so that they become less acidogenic.

5. Immunoglobulin A (IgA) molecules are secreted by plasma cells within the salivary glands, while another protein component is produced in the epithelial cells lining the ducts. The total concentration of IgA in saliva may be inversely related to caries experience.

6. Salivary proteins could increase the thickness of the acquired pellicle and so help to retard the movement of calcium and phosphate ions out of enamel.

Whilst there is no doubt that saliva possesses all the anti-caries properties listed above, research workers have been frustrated in their attempts to relate directly any particular salivary factor to the incidence of caries. One of the reasons for their failure is the fact that caries is a process occurring intermittently, in which host, microorganisms, and substrate are all involved. Since saliva has the ability to affect all of them in several different ways, it becomes easy to understand the difficulties encountered in trying to evaluate any single anti-caries factor at any one time. Nevertheless, there is sufficient evidence to demonstrate a negative correlation between buffering capacity of stimulated and unstimulated whole saliva and caries. In addition, there is no doubt that when saliva is absent, or drastically reduced in quantity, caries can be rampant. Hence caries preventive measures must be taken when there is any interference in salivary function which diminishes flow and when buffering capacity is low.

5.4.2 Radiation caries[3]

Following radiotherapy for tumours in the vicinity of the salivary glands or chemotherapy with cytotoxic drugs, conditions conducive to a rapid onset of caries are created not only by the shortage of saliva but also by the resultant dietary change. Liquids and soft foods, high in carbohydrate content are often consumed at frequent intervals throughout the day. To make matters worse there is also an alteration in the oral flora in favour of cariogenic organisms such as mutans streptococci and lactobaccilli as well as Candida[4] which can exacerbate the mucositis caused by the irradiation. If no special preventive regime is followed, rampant caries is very likely to develop.

It is now known that X-radiation in the doses administered in cancer therapy does not physically alter enamel to increase its caries susceptibility. Indeed, laboratory studies have demonstrated that irradiated enamel is more resistant than non-irradiated enamel to an artificial caries attack or demineralization. It has also been shown *in vivo* that teeth are only severely affected if the main salivary glands are within the radiation field so that there is a drastic reduction in saliva flow.

The typical pattern of caries development is shown in Figs. 1.7 (p. 9) and 5.1. The incisal edges of anterior teeth and the cusp tips of posterior teeth, which are normally very resistant to carious attack, suffer rapid destruction. The cervical margins of the teeth are also highly susceptible. All these areas are covered by only a thin layer of enamel so that, without the protection of saliva, caries rapidly invades dentine. If any root surfaces are exposed they are even more rapidly attacked and are very difficult to restore. It is very important that caries is controlled, because extractions can result in osteoradionecrosis or 'bone death' caused by radiation. This is due to a reduction in the osteocyte population and in the vascularity of the bone. Such changes make the bone vulnerable to trauma and infection, and impair its capacity to remodel and repair after extractions.

5.4.3 Management of dentate patients following radiotherapy for head and neck cancers

A regime to control caries and periodontal disease is vital in order to avoid the need for extractions. Salivary flow is diminished, particularly during the first year, increasing the risk of caries and the periodontium has lowered biological potential for healing.

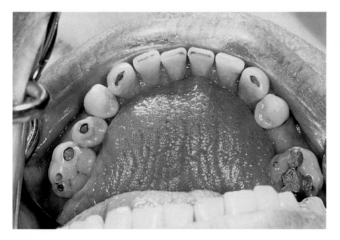

Fig. 5.1. A typical pattern of carious attack in a patient with xerostomia, in this case caused by radiotherapy in the region of the salivary glands. The cusp tips and incisal edges are typically attacked because dentine is often exposed by tooth wear in these areas. Dentine is more susceptible to caries than enamel.

For periondontal disease

It is essential to maintain healthy periodontal tissues since they offer a route for infection to the bone. Patients should therefore be monitored closely every three to four months when oral hygiene instruction is reinforced and scaling carried out when necessary. This emphasis on oral hygiene will also aid caries control.

For caries

Several studies show that, without dietary restrictions, caries can be successfully controlled by daily five-minute self-applications of a 1 per cent sodium fluoride gel in custom-made applicator trays. However, this level of commitment is difficult to achieve. When patients do not comply fully with such a regime, caries is uncontrolled, particularly where both parotids have been irradiated. Fortunately a simpler regime is now possible because of the availability of the antibacterial agent *chlorhexidine* which is an effective plaque inhibitor and anti-caries agent (see Section 8.5). Studies combining the use of fluoride and chlorhexidine have been successful in caries control after radiotherapy.[5,6] Based on the results of these studies, the following simple strategies are recommended:

1. Until salivary flow returns to normal limits, the risk of caries is high. Therefore, stimulated flow rates should be measured every three to four months to help to establish the level of caries risk (see Section 4.4.6).
2. Rigid dietary control is impractical. However, each time the patient is seen, the opportunity should be taken to reinforce the importance of avoiding sweet drinks and snacks. The pre-bed sweet drink is particularly dangerous. Taste sensation is lost during radiotherapy but when this returns two to four months later there often is a sudden craving for sweet foods and drinks. Patients should also be discouraged from attempts to stimulate salivary flow by sucking sweets. Instead, chewing a sugar-free gum containing xylitol will be safer and more effective. The use of a saliva substitute until salivary flow returns will also be helpful.
3. Patients should use a sodium fluoride (0.05 per cent NaF) mouthrinse daily for several years to help arrest any initial carious lesions. It will also help to alleviate sensitivity from pre-existing areas of exposed dentine which have lost the protective action of saliva. A low-alcohol or water-based product which does not contain alcohol should be chosen (see Section 7.7.2).
4. A 1 per cent chlorhexidine gel (Corsodyl) should be applied by the patient in custom-made applicator trays (Fig. 5.2) for five minutes every night for 14 days (see Section 8.5.2). This is repeated every three

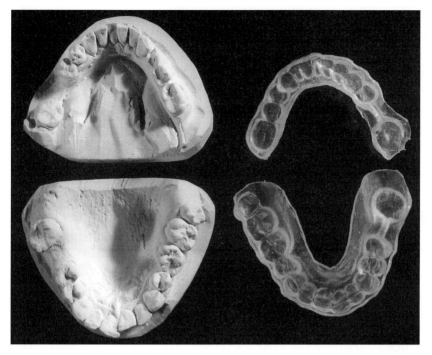

Fig. 5.2. Custom-made flexible, vacuum-moulded trays for self-application of chlorhexidine or fluoride gel.

to four months until salivary flow returns to normal. Such treatment has been shown to keep the level of mutans streptococci in control for at least three months.[6] Compliance with this regime can be checked before and after treatments by use of proprietary kits to measure levels of mutans streptococci (see Section 4.4.6). Any possible chlorhexidine staining can be removed when these patients are seen at their regular recall visits.

5. Chlorhexidine incorporated in a varnish (see Section 8.4.1) is currently being tested for its anti-caries action. If the results prove positive, the application of the chlorhexidine varnish in the dental chair could replace application of the gel by the patient.

5.4.4 Preventive measures for patients with dry mouths

The same fundamental steps that have to be taken before putting into practice any preventive measures also apply to these patients. The dentist must first recognize that a patient is 'at risk' (see Section 4.4); the situation must be explained to the patient and the patient must then be encouraged to adopt the following necessary preventive measures.

Dietary control

To alleviate the dryness in their mouths, these patients are tempted to suck sweets or drink sweet drinks at frequent intervals. It is therefore particularly important that following a diet analysis (see Section 6.6) dietary advice (see Section 6.7) is given. Particular attention should be given to the restriction of refined carbohydrate to mealtimes and avoiding the pre-bed sweet drink. The use of sugar-free chewing gum should be encouraged.

The use of fluoride

A daily sodium fluoride (0.05 per cent NaF) mouthwash should be recommended in the long term together with topical application of a fluoride varnish on any vulnerable sites by the dentist every six months.

Chlorhexidine gel application

When the shortage of saliva is not severe, dietary control and the use of fluoride may be the only measures required. In extreme cases chlorhexidine gel application every three to four months as outlined for radiotherapy patients is also necessary.

Without constant vigilance and regular monitoring by the dentist, a short lapse by the patient may have disastrous results.

REFERENCES

1. Thylstrup, A. and Fejerskov, O. (1994). *Textbook of cariology*, (2nd edn), Ch. 2: Saliva. Munksgaard, Copenhagen.
2. Edgar, W.M. and O'Mullane, D.M. (1990). *Saliva and dental health*. British Dental Journal, London.
3. Joyston-Bechal, S. (1992). Management of oral complications following radiotherapy. *Dent. update*, **19**, 232–8.
4. Brown, L. R., Dreizen, S., Handler, S., and Johnston, D. A. (1975). Effect of radiation-induced xerostomia on human oral microflora. *J. Dent. Res.*, **54**, 740–50.
5. Katz, S. (1982). The use of fluoride and chlorhexidine for the prevention of radiation caries. *J. Am. Dent. Assoc.*, **104**, 164–70.
6. Joyston-Bechal, S., Hayes, K., Davenport, E., and Hardie, J.M. (1992). Caries, mutans streptococci and lactobacilli in irradiated patients during a 12 month programme using chlorhexidine and fluoride. *Caries Res.*, **26**, 384–90.

6

Diet and caries

6.1 ACID PRODUCTION IN DENTAL PLAQUE

Fermentable carbohydrate and a cariogenic plaque need to be present on a tooth surface for acid to form. The acid is produced by bacterial metabolism of the carbohydrate substrate. The process is well illustrated by the Stephan curves shown in Fig. 1.1 (p. 4). This figure illustrates that the resting pH attained can vary with the tooth surface under test. Thus plaque within active occlusal carious cavities has a lower resting pH value than plaque on inactive occlusal carious lesions or sound surfaces. Similarly, following the sucrose rinse, the plaque within an active cavity shows the greatest fall in pH and remains low for longest. This demonstrates the relevance of operative dentistry in caries control and will be referred to again in Chapter 11.

Thus a single sucrose rinse, lasting a matter of seconds, can cause demineralization lasting between 20 minutes and several hours. Many factors determine the shape of the Stephan curve. The gradual return of pH to baseline values is a result of acids diffusing out of the plaque. In addition buffers in the plaque and salivary film exert a neutralizing effect. Saliva is very important in countering pH drops and this is one reason why people with dry mouths are at high risk to active caries. It also explains how stimulation of saliva can help to counteract a pH fall.

There has been a vast amount of experimental work linking fermentable carbohydrate and dental caries.[1-3] This work has proved that sugar is the most important dietary item in caries aetiology and it has shown how dietary advice has an important role in the management of the carious process.

6.2 SOME EVIDENCE LINKING DIET AND CARIES

The evidence linking diet and dental caries has been taken from epidemiological studies, human clinical studies, animal experiments, and plaque pH studies.

6.2.1 Epidemiological evidence

The consumption of sugar in substantial amounts is a recent trend in many areas of the world. Evidence linking sugar and caries has come from communities whose caries status has been recorded before and after an increase in the availability of sugar. One of the best known examples of this is the dental status of the inhabitants of Tristan da Cuhna, a remote rocky island in the South Atlantic. Their dental state was excellent in the 1930s when their diet comprised potatoes and other vegetables, meat, and fish. However, after 1940, there was a sharp increase in the consumption of imported sugary foods and a commensurate increase in caries.

The severe dietary restrictions in many countries during World War II were accompanied by a decrease in dental caries. The teeth which had already erupted showed the same reduced caries score as the developing teeth and the improvement was therefore due to a local dietary effect rather than a systemic nutritional one.

Epidemiological studies on other groups of people eating low amounts of sugar have also yielded interesting results. In 1942 an eccentric, wealthy Australian businessman transformed a spacious country mansion, called 'Hopewood House', into a home for young children of low socioeconomic background. When the children were 12 years old they could move to other accommodation but remained associated with the House. Since this entrepreneur attributed his own improvement in health to a drastic change in dietary habits, he stipulated that the children should be raised on a natural diet excluding refined carbohydrates. The dental surveys revealed a very low prevalence and severity of dental caries, much lower than in children of the same age and socioeconomic background attending ordinary state schools in New South Wales. However, after 12 years of age, when close supervision ended, their caries rate became virtually the same as that in the children in the state schools. This indicates that the diet eaten up to the age of 12 years did not confer any subsequent protection.

Another piece of evidence linking diet and caries concerns the rare hereditary disease fructose intolerance, which is caused by an inborn error of metabolism. Patients with this disease lack a certain liver enzyme and ingestion of foods containing fructose or sucrose causes severe nausea. Consequently they avoid these foods. The caries experience of these patients is very low, indicating that a group of people who are not able to tolerate many sugary foods are unlikely to develop much caries.

6.2.2 Interventional human clinical studies

An interventional study is one that measures the effects of altering, or intervening, in the study conditions in some way. In the dental field perhaps the most famous of all human clinical studies was begun in 1939 when the Swedish Government requested an investigation into 'What measures should be taken to reduce the frequency of the most common dental disease in Sweden?'. This led to a study on the relationship between diet and dental caries which was carried out at the Vipeholm Hospital, an institution for mentally defective individuals. The hospital, with its large number of permanent patients, provided an opportunity for a longitudinal study under well controlled conditions. A comparable study on human subjects will probably never be repeated as it would now be regarded as unethical to alter diets experimentally in directions likely to increase caries.

The patients were divided into one control and six experimental groups. Four meals were eaten daily and for one year patients received a diet relatively low in sugar with no sugar between meals. During this time the number of new carious lesions was assessed and found to be very low. Subsequently, the effect on caries of dietary changes involving the addition of large sucrose supplements in sticky or non-sticky form, either with or between meals, was assessed.

The control group, who continued with the basic diet, showed little increase in caries throughout the study. In the experimental groups the diet was supplemented by sucrose drinks or sucrose in bread or chocolate or caramels or 8 toffees or 24 toffees per day. There was a marked increase in caries in all groups except when the sucrose drink was taken at meal-times. The risk of sugar increasing the caries activity was greatest if the sugar was taken between meals, in a sticky form. Indeed, in the 24-toffee group, when the toffees were eaten between meals, the increase in caries was so great that the sugar supplement was withdrawn. This resulted in a fall in caries increment.

Dentists now base much of their dietary advice on the results of this study, stressing that the frequency of sugar intake should be reduced to confine sugar to mealtimes as far as possible. They advise against sticky, sweet foods and maintain that the rate of development of new disease will fall if this dietary advice is followed.

Another large-scale and important experiment on caries in humans was carried out in Turku, Finland, the aim being to compare the cario-genicity of sucrose, fructose, and xylitol. Xylitol is a sugar alcohol which is sweet but is not metabolized to acid by plaque microorganisms. The results of the study showed that both sucrose and fructose were cario-genic but the almost total substitution of sucrose by xylitol resulted in a substantial reduction in caries incidence. This introduces the concept that it may be possible to substitute sucrose by substances which will impart sweetness but are not cariogenic. This is covered in more detail in Section 6.7.2.

6.2.3 Non-interventional human studies

A non-interventional study relies on measurement alone without any active intervention in the study conditions. There have been a number of cross-sectional surveys of populations in which investigators have attempted to relate dietary habits to the prevalence of caries. Information about dietary habits is gathered by questionnaires and the caries data by clinical examination to obtain the DMF data. However, the latter represents a lifetime's caries experience and this may not correspond to 'snapshot' dietary diaries. Although some studies showed significant relationships between the amount and frequency of sugar intake and caries status, other studies did not.

Recently two longitudinal (two- and three-year) studies of adolescent schoolchildren living in communities with minimal fluoride in the drinking water were conducted in Northumberland, UK,[4] and Michigan, USA.[5] Multiple dietary histories were recorded and related to the caries that developed over the same time period. The correlations between the caries increments and dietary factors were positive but low. However, when the caries increments of children with the highest and lowest sugar intakes were compared obvious differences emerged. This would seem to show that with the current epidemiological picture of a decreased caries prevalence, dietary advice should be targeted at the high-risk group.

6.2.4 Animal experiments

The most commonly used animal in caries experiments is the rat, but hamsters, mice, and monkeys have also been used. One of the most important animal experiments was reported in 1954, when a system for rearing rats under germ-free conditions was devised. When these rats, who had no bacteria in their mouths, were fed a cariogenic diet, caries did not develop. This showed that a cariogenic oral microflora is essential for the development of dental caries.

Subsequently, the importance of the local effect of diet in the mouth was demonstrated when animals fed a cariogenic diet via a stomach tube did not develop the disease. Rat experiments have also confirmed the positive correlation between frequency of sugar intake and caries severity.

Animal experiments are commonly used to compare the cariogenicity of foods. Such work has shown that sucrose, glucose, fructose, galactose, lactose, and maltose are all cariogenic in varying degrees with sucrose being the most cariogenic.

Animal experiments on the cariogenicity of starch have yielded conflicting results showing starch products with a cariogenicity ranging from very low to comparable to that of glucose! Heating at temperatures used in cooking and baking causes a partial degradation of starch so it is possible that cooked starch may be capable of fermentation to acid in the mouth and this has been confirmed by plaque pH studies (see Section 6.2.5).

Experiments on rats have produced some interesting results when the animals were fed potato crisps. In the rat, which eats very frequently, some types of flavoured crisps cause caries. Crisps had long been regarded by dentists as a 'safe' snack and they are certainly less harmful than sweets. The eating pattern of man does not mimic the frequency of intake of the rat, so the results of this experiment should obviously be interpreted carefully. However, crisps should probably not be recommended as a safe snack, mainly because their high salt and fat content may be detrimental to the cardiovascular system.

6.2.5 Plaque pH studies

The measurement of plaque pH before, during, and after food is eaten should be a guide to the cariogenic potential of a food. Plaque pH can be measured intraorally by indwelling electrodes or extraorally on plaque samples harvested from the teeth. In these experiments Stephan curves (see Section 1.2.2) can be produced by plotting plaque pH against time. Snack foods and drinks have been ranked according to the value of the minimum pH reached by the plaque. This means that information is now available to enable dentists to advise patients which snacks are likely to be cariogenic, which may be harmless, and which may be positively beneficial.

Some snacks, like boiled sweets, sugared tea and coffee, and other sugared drinks clearly depress the pH. On the other hand some snacks, notably cheese and peanuts, and sugarless chewing gum actually tend to raise plaque pH, particularly if they are consumed after an acidogenic snack.

Plaque pH studies have also been used to differentiate between the potential cariogenicity of different sugars. Sucrose, glucose, fructose, and maltose appear to be of similar acidogenicity, while lactose and galactose produce less severe pH falls. Cow's milk (containing lactose) and unsugared tea with milk cause slight plaque pH falls, but cow's milk has only a very weak cariogenic potential.

Starch products, especially heat-degraded starch, have also been shown to have an acidogenic potential. Thus starch snacks cannot be considered to be completely safe for teeth.

6.3 SUGAR SUPPLIES IN THE UNITED KINGDOM

Figure 6.1 shows the daily *per capita* national estimates of sugar supplies in the UK from 1850 to 1987.[6] The drop in supplies during the two World

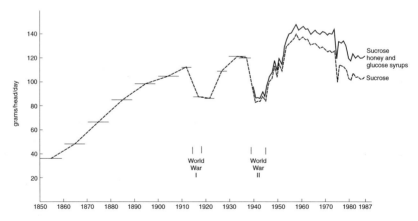

Fig. 6.1.   Supplies of selected sugars since 1850 expressed as grams per head of the population per day.[6]

Wars is obvious as are the rises following each. From the low point during World War II supplies of sucrose plus honey and glucose rose and peaked in 1958 when they averaged 147.5 g per head per day. Since 1974 supplies per head have fallen and in 1987 stood at approximately 120 g per head per day. Thus every man, woman, and child eats approximately 840 g of sugar per week. It will be obvious that these arithmetic means conceal enormous individual variation.

6.4 CULTURAL AND SOCIAL PRESSURES

Vast capital sums are invested in the sugar industry and related industries manufacturing soft drinks and confectionery. Large sums of money are also spent advertising sugar products, and the public are constantly exhorted to purchase sweet food products which they are told provide instant energy. Sweets are placed next to check-outs in supermarkets and school tuck shops and chocolate-bearing grannies flourish. In addition, many foods which are not generally thought of as cariogenic contain significant amounts of sucrose (sometimes called[6] 'hidden sugar'), for example, tomato soup, mustard, tomato sauce, frozen peas, tinned pasta, breakfast cereals, fruit yoghurts, many savoury baby foods, and rusks.

6.5 THE COMA REPORT[6]

In 1986 the Committee on Medical Aspects of Food Policy convened a Panel to inquire into and report on the health aspects of the consumption of sugars in United Kingdom diets. The report they produced is know as the COMA report. The following summary was produced by the Health Education Authority:

Sugar consumption rose steadily in the United Kingdom, peaking in 1958, and falling somewhat to the present day. The increasing use of sugar has been accompanied by claims that it is responsible for a number of diseases. The COMA Panel on Dietary Sugars considered the evidence for and against a role for sugars in the development of these diseases, and made appropriate recommendations.

The Panel described three main categories of sugars: 1. Instrinsic (part of cells in the food). 2. Milk sugars (the main sugars in milk and milk products). 3. Non-milk extrinsic sugars (including table sugar (sucrose), and glucose syrup).

They concluded that experience of tooth decay is positively related to the frequency and amount of non-milk extrinsic sugars consumption. Staple starchy foods, intrinsic and non-milk sugars are negligible causes of decay. They recommended that the consumption of non-milk extrinsic sugars should be decreased, and replaced in the diet by fresh fruit, vegetable and starchy foods.

Sugars contain roughly four kilocalories in every gram (compared with 9 kilo-calories from one gram of fat), but contain no other nutrients. Concern has been expressed that sugars might 'dilute' other nutrients in the diet. The Panel concluded that this is only likely to be a problem in people who are on low food intakes, and these people need to select their foods carefully to ensure an adequate intake of nutrients such as minerals and vitamins. Groups of people on low intakes might include, for example, the elderly or those on slimming diets.

As far as the development of obesity is concerned, the Panel said that this results from an excess intake of energy (kilocalories). Sugars may contribute to that total excess intake, but although they *might* favour overconsumption of food, the evidence which is currently available is insufficient to establish a link with obesity.

Reduction of non-milk extrinsic sugars along with restriction in fat intake, can help those who wish to lose weight.

The Panel concluded that there was no evidence for a direct link between sugar intake and the development of either non-insulin dependent diabetes or coronary heart disease. Any indirect link would be through an association with obesity.

They also said that there was no convincing evidence of a link between consumption of sugar and abnormal behaviour, and that no metabolic effects are likely within the current range of sugar intakes in the United Kingdom.

The main recommendations are for a reduction in the frequency and amount of consumption of non-milk extrinsic sugars; increased nutrition education for vulnerable groups; the increased availability of 'sugar free' medicines and development of 'low sugar' alternatives to sugar rich products; inclusion of nutrition in the training of health professionals; labelling of food with total sugars content; monitoring of sugar intakes; and further research in some areas.

6.6 DIET ANALYSIS[7,8]

The practical problems of diet analysis and advice in the caries-prone patient should be tackled systematically. Initially, the patient's current diet should be determined because if sensible advice is to be given this baseline information is needed. Dietary analysis should be carried out on all patients with a high caries activity and in those with an unusual caries pattern.

There are two principal techniques for determining food intake. One is to record the dietary intake during the preceding 24 hours, the so-called 24-hour recall system. This involves careful history taking and relies on the patient's memory and honesty. The other method is to obtain a three to four day written diet record, the patient recording food and liquid intake as it is consumed. This relies on the patient's full cooperation as well as honesty.

Both forms of diet recording suffer from the disadvantage that the record may not be representative of the diet consumed over a much longer time, although it is this which is likely to have been responsible for the caries and restoration status with which the patient presents. Thus, a diet history is an unscientific tool and must be interpreted with caution.

6.6.1 Recording the diet

The authors use a diet sheet as shown in Fig. 6.2. When this is given to patients it is explained that their help is needed to find the cause of their dental decay. The cause is related to what they eat and drink and for this reason it is necessary for them to record everything eaten and drunk over a four-day period, together with the time of eating. (In addition, any medication should be entered.) They are requested to keep the diet sheet with them and fill it in at the time to avoid missing anything. Quantities of food consumed are not specifically requested but it should be stressed that nothing should be changed because a record is being kept. Dentist and patient are partners in the investigation and the object of the exercise is to help, not to condemn.

Although this strategy is useful for many patients, it may be inappropriate for others. Sometimes variable dietary habits will mean that the four-day record is inappropriate or even misleading. Shift workers may have different dietary habits from week to week, as may those whose work neces-

Diet Analysis

	THURSDAY		FRIDAY		SATURDAY		SUNDAY	
	Time	Item	Time	Item	Time	Item	Time	Item
BEFORE BREAKFAST								
Breakfast								
MORNING								
Mid-day meal								
AFTERNOON								
Evening meal								
EVENING and NIGHT								

Fig. 6.2.   A form on which a patient may record diet over a four-day period. This has been designed to highlight the between-meal snack, thus facilitating patient education when the sheet is completed and returned. On the reverse side of the diet sheet there are simple instructions explaining how it should be filled in.

sitates frequent trips abroad. 'Bingers' will be unwilling to commit their usual dietary pattern to paper. A medical history may reveal unstable health conditions such as intermittent ulcer problems, and thus a four-day record may be inappropriate. However, if the patient understands the purpose of the record, he/she may suggest how best it is kept. For instance the shift worker may record two days on duty and two days off. Those with a medical history may record typical days when they are 'well' and other days when they are 'ill'. Finally it must be appreciated that a patient may not always tell the truth, although if the patient knows what to lie about, progress has been made!

6.6.2 Analysis of the dietary record

Once the patient returns the completed sheet dentist and patient can begin to look at it together. A highlighter pen is useful to mark items containing sugar. If the dentist encourages the patient to identify these it will become apparent whether the patient realizes which items are sweet.

The relevance of sugar and the role of bacterial plaque should be explained, and then the number of sugar attacks can be counted and this number recorded at the top of each day. This gives the dentist the opportunity to explain the relevance of frequency of sugar attacks. The amount of time the plaque remains acid and capable of causing demineralization varies depending on such factors as the consistency of the food, salivary flow, salivary clearance rates, and the activity of the carious lesion.

However, these complex and important scientific deliberations will be lost on the patient who needs a simple (but scientifically simplistic) message. It would not be unreasonable to suggest that after a sugar attack the plaque is likely to remain acid for one hour, thus eight attacks would equal eight hours of acid plaque.

Special note is taken of:

(1) the main meals, to see whether they are sufficiently substantial. This is important to prevent the patient craving food in-between meals;
(2) the between-meal snacks. Are they cariogenic?
(3) any medication, particularly if it is based on a sucrose syrup or if it is likely to cause dry mouth or thirst;
(4) the number and type of between-meal drinks. Are these cariogenic?
(5) the consistency of any between-meal snacks. Are they sticky and therefore take a long time to clear from the mouth?
(6) the use of sucrose-containing chewing gum or any sweet that takes a long time to dissolve in the mouth;
(7) any sugary pre-bed snacks or drinks.

Figures 6.3–6.5 show examples of diet analysis sheets. Figure 6.3 is one day from a diet sheet kept by a 24-year-old mechanical engineer referred to a consultant from a practitioner because of a high caries rate. The patient was an intelligent young man, concerned about his teeth and grateful for all his dentist was doing for him. The mouth was clean and well restored but white spot lesions were developing around the margins of restorations and the dentist's radiographs, taken at yearly intervals showed approximal enamel lesions were progressing into dentine. The diet sheet shows ten separate sugar attacks, including a sugary drink just before bed. The patient ate frequently and used the term 'grazing' to describe his eating habits. All drinks were cariogenic and the main meals were inadequate because he ate as he worked.

The diet sheet in Fig. 6.4 is from a middle aged secretary with a high incidence of caries. This patient returned to the surgery after having kept the record, saying that she now realized the cause of the decay in her mouth. In addition she said how surprised she was to see how little she ate at mealtimes.

DIET ANALYSIS

		THURSDAY
	Time	10 attacks Item 1 pre-bed
BEFORE BREAK-FAST	7.15	1 pint skimmed milk milk shake
Breakfast	8.30	Black coffee + Sugar
MORNING	10.00 / 12.00	White coffee + Sugar 2 cheese rolls Bag Crisps, Cake Twix White coffee + Sugar
Mid-day Meal	13.30	2 cheese rolls Cake 1 mint Apple
AFTER-NOON	15.30 / 17.00	White coffee + Sugar Tea + Sugar 4 Biscuits
Evening Meal	19.30	Pizza Ribena Ice Cream
EVENING	21.30 / 22.30	Glass of coke Glass of coke

Fig. 6.3. One day in the initial diet sheet of a 24-year-old mechanical engineer.

DIET ANALYSIS (See notes on other side) ✻ = 2 spoons of sugar.

	THURSDAY		FRIDAY		SATURDAY		SUNDAY	
	Time	Item	Time	Item	Time	Item	Time	Item
BEFORE BREAKFAST	7.45	Tea ✻	7.00	Tea ✻	7.00	Tea ✻		
Breakfast	9.00	Coffee ✻	8.45	Coffee ✻	10.00	Tea ✻ 2 pieces of toast		
MORNING	10.00 / 10.45	Coffee ✻ Roll and butter / Coffee ✻	9.30 / 10.45 / 11.45	Coffee ✻ Roll and butter Coffee ✻ / Coffee ✻	11.00 / 12.00	Coffee ✻ / Coffee ✻	10.45 / 11.30	Tea ✻ / Tea ✻
Mid-day Meal	12.30 / 1.30	Coffee ✻ / Coffee ✻	1.45	Cheese & onion Sandwich ½ lager	1.0	Coffee ✻ 1 muesli biscuit	2.0	Beef roast potatoes Carrots : greens fresh pear Tea ✻
AFTERNOON	2.30 / 3.45 / 4.15	Coffee ✻ / Coffee ✻ / Coffee ✻	2.30 / 3.15 / 4.00 / 5.00	Coffee ✻ / Coffee ✻ / Coffee ✻ / Coffee ✻	3.00 / 4.15	Tea ✻ / Tea ✻	3.30	Tea ✻
Evening Meal	7.30	Country hash Tea ✻	9.00	Lasagne Tea ✻	7.00	Spare Ribs, Rice Tea ✻	5.00 / 6.30	Tea ✻ / Coffee ✻
EVENING & NIGHT	9.00 / 10.30	2 muesli biscuits Tea ✻ Pear	10.00 / 11.15	Tea ✻ / Tea ✻ 2 biscuits	9.30 / 11.00	Tea ✻ / Tea ✻	8.00 / 10.00	Coffee ✻ Cheese & biscuit Tea ✻

Fig. 6.4. A diet sheet completed by a middle-aged secretary with a very high incidence of caries. This lady returned to the surgery saying that she now realized that drinking frequent cups of sweetened tea and coffee was the likely cause of her caries.

Figure 6.5 shows one day in a remarkable diet where the patient drank regularly every two hours, day and night. The relevant feature of this diet sheet was that the patient was taking chlorpromazine (Largactil), an antipsychotic drug, and lithium carbonate for depression. These drugs cause dry mouth and thirst respectively (see Chapter 5) and the patient was consequently continually drinking and many of these drinks were cariogenic. Unfortunately the remains of the dentition were beyond repair and the patient is now edentulous.

6.7 DIETARY ADVICE

On the basis of the diet analysis, the clinician may be in a position to indicate to the patient the constituents of the diet which may be harmful and to make some positive recommendations. Dietary advice should be tailored to the needs of the individual patient and should form part of a comprehensive preventive programme consisting of oral hygiene instruction, the use of topical fluoride preparations, and fissure sealants.

	THURSDAY	
	Time	*Item*
BEFORE BREAKFAST	6·50 7·12, 7·30	Lucozade Grapefruit juice Lucozade.
Breakfast	9·30	Cereal, milk, glucose, toast marmelade; Coffee with glucose
MORNING	10·15 11·05 12·20 1·00	Tablets Lithium Valium Lemon drink Guiness Tablets Lithium
Mid-day Meal	1·45	Macaroni Cheese Tomato Shortbread Biscuits Water.
AFTERNOON	2·40 3·40 4·35	Lemon drink, sugar & lemon juice water Tea and glucose Lemon drink.
Evening Meal	6·45	Omelete, potato Biscuits, raisins, water.
EVENING & NIGHT	8·10 8·45 9·45 9·55 10·05 1·10 3·30 5·30	Water Lime juice Peanuts: water Glacé cherry Tablets Lithium Valium Largactil Lucozade Lucozade Lucozade

Fig. 6.5. One day from an unusual diet sheet kept by a patient who was thirsty because of her medication and consequently drank regularly. Unfortunately most of the drinks were cariogenic.

6.7.1 General advice

Dietary advice must be practical, setting realistic goals (see Section 9.3.9). It is impossible to expect patients to cut sugar completely out of the diet but it is feasible to reduce the total amount of sugar consumed, and to restrict sugar intake mainly to mealtimes.

Sugary foods or drinks between meals are particularly harmful and should be avoided in the caries-prone patient. Crisps, peanuts, or cheese may be acceptable alternatives, although peanuts should not be given to children under five years as there is a real risk of death due to asphyxiation following inhalation of a single nut. The bed-time snack or drink is particularly important since salivary flow is virtually absent at night and plaque pH may remain low for many hours.

It is neither necessary nor practical to stop children eating sweets altogether. However, it is not unreasonable to suggest that they are restricted to one day a week. In any case, children should be encouraged to eat a balanced meal before any sweets are given. If sweets are eaten, they will do least damage as part of a main meal. Grannie's advice of 'Don't eat them all at once' as she hands over the chocolates could be disastrous for dental health.

Adults should also be advised not to eat sugary snacks between meals, but if sugary snacks are cut out of the diet the patient may be hungry and thus a list of sugar-free snacks and drinks (Table 6.1) is useful so that the patient may suggest a suitable alternative. However, it is often sweetened drinks that are the problem, and here sugar substitutes can be very helpful.

6.7.2 Sugar substitutes[2,9]

There is increasing interest in the use of sweetening agents which confer sweetness but are safer for teeth. They are useful because many people have a sweet tooth and thus when used to replace sugars in foods that are frequently consumed, such as sweet snacks, drinks, and liquid medicines, they will have dental benefits. These products may be divided into two categories: those which have no calorific value (non-nutritive or intense sweeteners) and those which have a calorific value (nutritive or bulk sweeteners). The non sugar sweeteners currently permitted in UK can be

Table 6.1 Sugar-free snacks and drinks[7]

Do you find it hard to think up snacks and drinks that are safe for teeth? The following are some examples of alternatives to confectionery and sugar based drinks. It is not intended to be a fully comprehensive list but rather a rough guide to show that these days there is a wide selection of alternatives to be found on supermarket shelves that will not harm teeth in between meals. By reading food labels and using a little imagination you will no doubt find many more. Look at labels carefully, and beware of the following: sucrose, glucose, fructose, dextrose, glucose syrup, honey, corn syrup, invert sugar syrup, molasses, treacle, maltose. These are all sugary types of products and can damage the teeth. Brown sugar is just as bad as white!

Drinks

Water
Tea and coffee without
sugar
Milk: Children under 5
should be given whole
milk not skimmed or
semi-skimmed. The
following drinks are all
sugar free and will not
cause decay but it
should be remembered
that as with any fruit
drinks, they are acidic
and if drunk to excess,
can dissolve the surface
of the teeth. For example:

Kia-ora whole orange
drink
Robinson's Special
R Fruit juice drinks
Supermarkets' own
brands: check labels
Diet Lemonade, Diet Cola
Diet Pepsi, Diet 7 Up

The sweetening agent in
these will be one of the
artificial sweeteners
like aspartame, saccharin,
acesulfame-K.

Snacks

Toast
Rolls
Sandwiches
Pitta bread
French bread
Cheese scones
Cornish wafers (Jacob's)
Cream crackers (Jacob's,
Sainsbury, Tesco)
Butter puffs (Crawford's)
Twiglets
Crunchy stick (Tesco)
Wotsits
Hula Hoops
Crisps: various assorted,
check labels if unsure.
Low fat and low salt
crisps are also available.
Crisp rolls (in pre-
packaged bags from
supermarkets)

Fillings/toppings for sandwiches, rolls

Meat and fish spreads
Cold meat
Eggs
Tinned fish
Marmite: not suitable before
6 months of age
Bovril: not suitable before
6 months of age
Peanut butter: sugar free, e.g.
Whole Earth
Original Crunchy
Cheese: low fat is available
Kraft Dairylea cheese slices
Delight low fat diary cheese
slices
Sun-Pat medium cheddar
spread
Laughing Cow low fat Dairy
Spread

Raw fruits and vegetables

Fruit is sweet and not
surprisingly contains sugars.
Although not sugar free, it is
a good alternative to biscuits or
cakes, which are high in sugar.
Apples, oranges, pears,
bananas, etc.
Carrots, celery, radish, etc.
Nuts: not suitable before
5 years of age
N.B. Dried fruit (e.g. raisins,
sultanas) is high in sugar and
therefore not a safe snack.
Muesli bars—often sold as
health snacks—are often high
in dried fruits, honey, glucose
syrup and sugar and are
therefore potentially harmful
to teeth.

Yogurts

St Ivel Shape
Marks and Spencer Lite
Tesco Healthy Eating very
low fat
Boots Shapers
The sweetening agent in these
products will be aspartame or
aspartame and acesulfame-K.

Sweets

Chewing gum: various sugar
free
Trebor Sugar Free Coolmints

Alternative sweeteners in tablet and granule form

Aspartame:
(Nutra Sweet)
Canderel Spoonful
Canderel tablets
Boots Shapers Granulated
Sweetener
Boots Shapers tablets

Aspartame and
acesulfame-K:
Hermesetas 'New Taste'
tablets
Hemesetas Granulated
Sweetener

Saccharin:
Hemesetas 'Original' tablets
Sweetex tablets
Natrena tablets

Aspartame and saccharin:
Sweetex granulated

Recommendations to help you and your family keep teeth healthy

1. Have 3 meals a day
   containing protein,
   green vegetables,
   salad, fruit,
   or cheese.

2. Discourage sugary
   snacks and drinks
   between meals; if you
   are really hungry or
   thirsty between meals
   try to choose 'safe'
   items.

3. Limit sugar intake to the
   3 meals because sugar
   does less harm to teeth if
   taken with meals. Give
   any sweets at the end of
   a meal. Damage to teeth
   occurs when sugar is
   spread out during the
   day, constantly attacking
   teeth.

seen in Table 6.2 together with a list of sugars or substances containing sugar. This list should be useful when helping a patient to examine food labels to see if the constituents are potentially cariogenic.

Non-nutritive sweeteners

These are sometimes called 'intense sweeteners' because they have a sweetness many times that of sucrose. These substances impart sweetness but furnish no calories. They are safe for teeth because they cannot act as an energy source for dental plaque microorganisms and acid cannot be derived from them.

The three non-nutritive sweeteners readily available in the United Kingdom are saccharin, acesulfame-K and aspartame. They are produced in both tablet and granule form (Fig. 6.6). Saccharin was discovered more than a century ago and has been used as a sweetener in foods and drinks for over 80 years. It is 300 times as sweet as sugar weight for weight but suffers the disadvantage of a bitter, metallic aftertaste which some consumers find unacceptable. For some years its safety was debated because bladder tumours were found in male rats fed on exceptionally high doses of saccharin. However, saccharin has been found to be safe, even at very high levels, for human consumption.

Acesulfame-K is chemically related to saccharin but has an improved aftertaste. Aspartame (trade names Canderel, Nutra Sweet) is a slightly different product containing two amino acids. Its taste is regarded as the closest to that of sucrose with no bitterness.

Ideally these various sweeteners should be kept in the surgery (Fig. 6.6) so that tea or coffee can be made sweetened with these various alternatives

Table 6.2 Sweeteners

Sugar or sugar containing	Sugar substitutes	
	Non-nutritive	Nutritive
Sucrose	Saccharin	Sorbitol
Glucose	Acesulfame-K	Mannitol
Glucose syrup	Aspartame	Xylitol
Fructose	Thaumatin	Lacitol
Sorbose		Hydrogenated glucose syrup
Lactose		Isomalt
Maltose		
Dextrose		
Honey		
Corn syrup		
Invert sugar syrup		
Molasses		
Treacle		

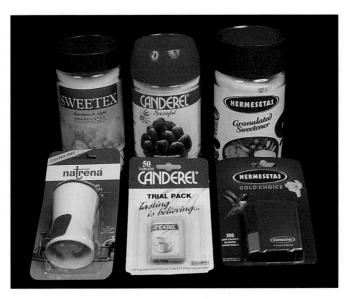

Fig. 6.6. Artificial sweeteners in tablet and granule form.

and the patient invited to taste and rank them for acceptability (see Section 9.3.8). It is our subjective impression that patients vary in what they find acceptable, and we have certainly found patients (and dental students) who cannot distinguish the sugar substitute from sugar!

These artificial sweeteners are also used in the manufacture of several drinks (Table 6.1) and from a caries point of view, substitution of the artificially sweetened beverage may be helpful. However, it must be remembered that such drinks, although not cariogenic, are very acidic and may cause erosion if consumed frequently.

Nutritive sweeteners

The nutritive sweeteners are sugar alcohols and the most useful are sorbitol and xylitol. Mannitol, lactitol, hydrogenated glucose syrup, and isomalt are also approved for use in food products in UK. *Sorbitol* is found naturally in some fruits and berries but for economic reasons both sorbitol and *mannitol* are prepared industrially from glucose. Sorbitol is only about half as sweet as sucrose and relatively inexpensive. It is used in chewing gum, sugar-free sweets, 'diabetic' food products, sugar-free medicines, and toothpaste. Since it is only partially absorbed from the bowel, large amounts cause a laxative effect because of osmotic transfer of water into the bowel. Sorbitol is fermented by some plaque microorganisms but at a much slower rate than sucrose. There is a suggestion that with long-term use by humans the oral microflora will adapt and start to be able to convert it to acid so that it may not be completely safe for use in patients with dry mouths. However, it is regarded as much less cariogenic than sucrose. Drinks, sweets, and chewing gums containing sorbitol are likely to be safer for teeth than their sucrose-containing counterparts.

Xylitol is a sugar alcohol obtained commercially from birch trees, coconut shells, and cotton seed hulls. It is twice as expensive to produce as sorbitol and is ten times the cost of sucrose. Like sorbitol it has a laxative effect, but unlike sorbitol it cannot be fermented by oral microorganisms. Xylitol has an anticaries effect and it appears to do this by several different mechanisms. It stimulates salivary flow, enhances remineralization, and reduces the levels of mutans streptococci in the mouth. This makes it a very attractive agent to put in chewing gum where it may encourage salivary flow and reduce the cariogenic microflora.

Lactitol is a relative newcomer on the sugar alcohol scene. It is derived from lactose, has half the energy value of sucrose but is only a third as sweet as sucrose. It should be a valuable bulking agent in foods but may cause osmotic diarrhoea.

Hydrogenated glucose syrup (Lycasin) is obtained by enzymatic hydrolysis of corn starch. It is potentially very confusing that hydrogenated glucose syrup is sugar-free, whereas glucose syrup is basically a solution of glucose and cariogenic. Lycasin is the registered trade mark of hydrogenated glucose syrup and is used in confectionary and pharmaceutical products in several countries. It has less of a laxative effect than other sugar alcohols.

Isomalt (Palatinit) is a mixture of two disaccharide alcohols and is said to be particularly useful in the manufacture of sugar-free chocolate.

Toothfriendly sweets

A number of sweets are now available which have been scientifically tested and passed as safe for teeth. These are called toothfriendly sweets and these products carry a special logo (Fig. 6.7) known as the happy tooth symbol.

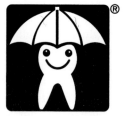

Fig. 6.7. The toothfriendly sweet logo.

This logo is a registered certification mark, controlled by an international and several national associations which operate on a non-profit making basis and are governed by the dental profession. There are Toothfriendly Associations in Germany, France, Belgium, and the United Kingdom.

The idea began in Switzerland in the 1960s when staff at Zurich Dental School developed a system for monitoring the pH of dental plaque while foods were being eaten. Sugary foods caused a sharp fall in plaque pH while foods sweetened with non-fermentable sweeteners did not depress plaque pH. This method became known as the intraoral plaque pH telemetry test and has become accepted, after extensive investigation, as a valid indicator of 'safe for teeth' foods.

In 1969, the Swiss Office of Health accepted that the test could identify foods with a low caries risk and allowed foods to be advertised as 'zahnschonend' or '*ménageant les dents*'. However, public awareness of the dental value of these products was low until 1982 when 'Aktion Zahnfreundlich' was formed as a joint venture between the Swiss University Dental Institutes and the confectionery industry. Aktion Zahnfreundlich (also known as the Sympadent Association) was legally registered as a non-profit-making association of dentists and producers of 'safe for teeth' confectionery. Against payment of royalty, members of the Sympadent Association obtain the right to use the happy tooth pictogram on wrappers of tested products. This income is then devoted to promoting the awareness of the benefits of these products to the general public. By 1991, consumer surveys showed that about 75 per cent of the Swiss population and nearly 90 per cent of Swiss children were fully aware of the significance of the happy tooth symbol. Today, around 80 per cent of chewing gum and 20 per cent of other confectionery sold in Switzerland carries the 'safe for teeth' logo.

The success of the Sympadent Association in Switzerland was noticed in neighbouring countries. In 1985, a similar scheme began in Germany, followed by France in 1990 and Belgium in 1992. Due to international sales, products carrying the Toothfriendly symbol can be seen in at least 20 countries, from Europe to South America and the Far East.

The test is based on the measurement of the pH of dental plaque, *in vivo*. The electrode used to monitor the plaque pH is built into a denture-like appliance which is worn by a volunteer subject. After standardization of the electrode, five volunteers eat the test product, and changes in the pH of dental plaque are monitored. If the pH in dental plaque does not fall below 5.7 during and for 30 minutes after consumption, and if at the same time the amount of potentially erosive food acids do not exceed a specified threshold value as measured by a plaque-free electrode, then the product passes the test and qualifies to carry the happy tooth logo.

For practical purposes, confectionery sweetened solely with non-sugar sweeteners and not containing fermentable carbohydrate or excessive amounts of acid is likely to pass the test. There are currently three recognized toothfriendly testing centres, in Zurich and Bern in Switzerland and Erfurt in Germany.

6.7.3 Protective foods

The consumption of some foods after sugar has been shown to raise plaque pH. Cheese is useful in this respect and can be recommended as the last course of a meal or as a 'safe' snack. Chewing gums containing xylitol have also been shown to raise salivary pH after a sugar snack.

6.7.4 'Safe' snacks

It is really remarkably difficult to draw up a list of snacks that are safe in all respects. Although cheese is safe for teeth its high saturated fat content may not please cardiologists. This group may be similarly concerned at the recommendation of plain crisps owing to their high salt and fat content. Fruit is less cariogenic than sweets but contains natural sugar. Dried fruits such as raisins and apricots have a high sugar content and cannot be considered as 'safe' snacks. Many fruits are very acid (lemons, sour apples, oranges, grapefruit) and excessive use of such fruits or their juices may cause acid erosion of the dental tissues. However, used in moderation, fruit is safer than sweets. Nuts are a safe snack for older children and adults.

Bread and unsweetened biscuits are relatively safe for teeth provided they are not spread with jam or honey. Some raw vegetables such as carrots and tomatoes are 'safe' but are not to everyone's taste. A list of sugar-free snacks and drinks should be used when giving dietary advice. Table 6.1 shows such a list, correct when we went to press, but as the years go by brand name products may change and their sugar content should be checked. Encourage patients to suggest their own solutions to problems, then write down the advice that has been agreed in the notes and in a legible form for the patient to take away. Figure 6.8 shows the list of suggestions drawn up with the 24-year-old mechanical engineer whose diet sheet is seen in Fig. 6.3. At the patient's next visit this list was discussed again to see which suggestions were realistic and therefore taken on board (see Section 9.3.10).

6.7.5 Advice to pregnant and nursing mothers

There is little evidence in modern societies that children suffer any dental abnormalities due to maternal malnutrition. Nor is there evidence to

SUGGESTIONS

1.	Aim 2–3 sugar attacks/day
2.	Never sugar before bed
3.	Coffee and tea—try no sugar
4.	If coke; use <u>diet</u> variety
5.	Water is safe (patient hates milk!)
6.	Try savory roll to eat at work
7.	Try to eat more lunch and reduce 'grazing'!
8.	Eat lots in evening
9.	Beer is not cariogenic!

Fig. 6.8. The written suggestions for dietary change given to the 24-year-old mechanical engineer whose diet sheet is seen in Fig. 6.3. Each suggestion has been discussed with the patient and agreed as 'worth a try'.

suggest there will be any significant benefit to the teeth from a pregnant woman eating additional minerals, vitamins, or fluoride. There is no apparent relationship between nutritional deficiencies during tooth formation and caries.

Breast feeding is strongly recommended by paediatricians since there is strong evidence that the number of infections and allergic conditions such as eczema are reduced in children who are breast fed, probably because of the antibodies present in human milk. From a cariogenic point of view it is widely believed that breast feeding is less harmful than bottle feeding. This may be because breast milk contains lactose which is significantly less cariogenic than sucrose. However, very rare cases of rampant caries have been described in infants breast feeding on true demand for up to two years or more (see p. 9). In this condition the infants suckle regularly through the day and the night, perhaps 60 times per 24 hour period for several years.

The practice of adding sugar or honey to baby foods should be discouraged since this may cause the development of a 'sweet tooth' and influence the selection of cariogenic foods in later life. The use of a sucrose vehicle for vitamin supplements is also unwise since these have been implicated in the aetiology of rampant caries in infants and young children. Above all, the child should never be given a dummy or bottle containing a sugar solution to be sucked at will, nor should a bottle of sweet drink be suspended in the cot so that the young child can drink at will throughout the night without waking the parent. This is likely to cause rampant caries (nursing-bottle caries) of the deciduous dentition (Fig. 1.8, p. 9).

6.7.6 Young children

Parents should be encouraged to give their children foods which do not foster a 'sweet' tooth. It is said that if children are given a savoury diet from an early age they will be happy to eat meals containing such foodstuffs in preference to sweet-tasting foods. Friends and relatives should be encouraged to bring small toys, fruit, or crisps as presents rather than sweets. Drinks at bedtime, other than water, should be strongly discouraged.

6.7.7 Chronically sick children

Many children with chronic medical disorders are placed at considerable risk when dental treatment procedures have to be carried out. Every care should be taken to prevent caries in such patients, although the syrupy vehicles often used to administer medicines make caries more likely. There is a need for strict dietary control as well as thorough oral hygiene, fluoride supplementation, and fissure sealing of susceptible teeth. Sugar-free medicines should be recommended.

6.7.8 Patients with dry mouths

This group is particularly at risk to dental caries as discussed in Chapter 5. Thirst or the need to lubricate the mouth often results in the consumption of frequent sweet drinks or the chewing and sucking of sweets. Mouth lubricants and/or 'safe' drinks and sugar-free chewing gums should be recommended.

6.7.9 Dietary changes

Diet may remain constant over many years, but the dentist should watch for changes in caries status, and if a patient starts to develop new lesions the dietary cause should be sought. Perhaps the patient has left home, gone to boarding school, or started work and changed his or her diet radically. Alternatively, retirement, bereavement, or illness may have resulted in changed dietary habits. Sometimes mints are substituted for cigarettes when giving up smoking and the mint habit may persist long after the craving for a cigarette has gone. Mints sweetened with xylitol would be safe for teeth.

6.7.10 Monitoring the effect of dietary advice

Food intake and dietary habits are very difficult to influence. To find out whether the patient has followed the suggested dietary recommendations, the dentist can simply ask the patient about any changes. However, it is probably better to ask the patient to fill in another diet sheet. Figure 6.9 is a subsequent diet sheet filled in by the 'grazing' mechanical engineer (Figs. 6.3 and 6.8) (see Section 9.3.10). It would appear that this highly motivated young man had done all that had been suggested.

DIET ANALYSIS

		THURSDAY	
	Time	2 attacks	Item
BEFORE BREAK-FAST	7.30		White coffee
Breakfast			
MORNING	10.00		2 cheese + salad rolls Crisps Cake White coffee
Mid-day Meal	13.00		2 cheese + salad rolls Apple
AFTER-NOON	15.30 17.00		Glass of Orange Cup of Tea
Evening Meal	18.00		Pizza Garlic Bread Salad
EVENING	21.00 23.00		Diet coke Beer

Fig. 6.9. One day in the second diet sheet produced by the 24-year-old mechanical engineer. Figure 6.3 shows the original diet sheet and Fig. 6.8 the suggestions for change agreed with the patient.

6.8 DIETARY MISCONCEPTIONS

A number of misconceptions exist about diet and dental caries and it may be appropriate to end this chapter by laying a few ghosts! One serious misconception is that only refined carbohydrates (sucrose or white sugar) are harmful to teeth while other carbohydrates are not. Sucrose is certainly regarded as the 'arch-criminal' because it is the most abundant sugar. It is used by food manufacturers all over the world as a food ingredient and it is readily used by bacteria to form extracelluar polysaccharides which make plaque thicker and stickier. However, other sugars, such as glucose, fructose, dextrose, glucose syrup, honey, corn syrup, invert sugar syrup, molasses, treacle, and maltose are also bad for teeth, although they may be somewhat less damaging than sucrose. In addition brown sugar is just as bad as white.

Health foods are very fashionable nowadays; it has been suggested that fibrous foods such as apples and carrots 'clean' teeth thus removing plaque and preventing caries. While fibrous foods are preferable to a sucrose snack, there is no evidence that they can 'clean' the teeth. Another popular health food is honey. This so-called 'natural' sugar food is just as cariogenic as other sugars. Many brands of muesli contain both sugar and honey. In the same way, the naturally occurring sugar in fruit juices makes these products just as cariogenic as the squashes.

Finally, it is very common for patients who are asked to give up sugar in tea and coffee to reduce the amount of sugar (say one teaspoon instead of two) rather than giving it up completely. Thus, the frequency of sugar intake and therefore the frequency of pH fall may not be altered. It is important to check that patients really understand the message, otherwise they may make a considerable effort to no avail (see p. 151).

REFERENCES

1. Murray, J.J. (1989). *The prevention of dental disease*, (2nd edn), Ch. 2: Diet and dental caries. Oxford University Press.
2. Rugg-Gunn, A.J. (1993). *Nutrition and dental health*. Oxford University Press.
3. Thylstrup, A. and Fejerskov, O (1994). *Textbook of clinical cariology*, (2nd edn), Ch. 13: Diet and the carious process. Munksgaard, Copenhagen.
4. Rugg-Gunn, A.J., Hackett, A.F., Appleton, D.R., Jenkins, G. N., and Eastoe, J.E. (1984). Relationship between dietary habits and caries increment assessed over two years in 405 English adolescent school children. *Arch. Oral Biol.*, **29**, 983–92.
5. Burt, B.A., Eklund, S.A. Morgan, K.J., Larkin, F.E., Guire, K.E., Brown, L.O., and Weintraub, J.A. (1988). The effects of sugar intake and the frequency of inges-

tion on dental caries increment in a three-year longitudinal study. *J. Dent. Res.*, **67**, 1422–9.

6. *Dietary sugars and human disease* (1989). Report of the Panel on Dietary Sugars. Committee on Medical Aspects of Food Policy. Her Majesty's Stationery Office, London.

7. Barker, T. (1994). Realistic dietary advice for patients. *Dent. Update*, **21**, 28–34.

8. Kidd E.A.M. (1995) The use of diet analysis and advice in the management of dental caries in adult patients. *Oper. Dent.* **20**, 86–93.

9. Grenby, T.H. (1991). Update on low-calorie sweeteners to benefit dental health. *Int. Dent. J.*, **41**, 217–24.

7

Fluoride supplementation in dental practice

7.1 INTRODUCTION

In 1901 an American dentist, Dr F. McKay, who had recently arrived in Colorado Springs from Pennsylvania, noticed that the teeth of many of his patients had a particular appearance which he called *mottled enamel*. He described this enamel as 'characterized by minute white flecks, or yellow or brown spots or areas, scattered irregularly or streaked over the surface of a tooth, or it may be a condition where the entire tooth surface is of a dead paper-white, like the colour of a china dish'.[1] It was not until the 1930s that excessive fluoride in the drinking water (>2.0 parts per million (ppm F) or 2 mg F/litre) was shown to be responsible for this mottling and the condition was related to a low prevalence of dental caries. This work was done in the USA[2] and Britain.[3] The term *dental fluorosis* was coined and research was begun to study the possible benefits of fluoride.

In 1942 Dean and his co-workers[4] published the classical epidemiological studies carried out by the US Public Health Service on children, 12–14 years of age, living in 20 towns, relating caries experience and the fluoride content of the water supply. They showed that when the drinking water contained about 1 ppm of fluoride the teeth of the lifelong inhabitants of that area had a low caries prevalence but no signs of dental fluorosis. For example, children aged 12–14 years had 50 per cent less caries than those with no fluoride in the water. These observations led to the addition of fluoride to fluoride-deficient water supplies in several controlled clinical studies throughout the world.[5] The optimum level of fluoride recommended in temperate climates was 1 ppm while in tropical climates, where water consumption was greater, the level was reduced to 0.7 ppm. The results of these studies showed conclusively that it was possible to reduce caries by supplying optimal levels of fluoride. Since the early studies it has become clear that in order to continue to benefit from fluoridated water, it must continue throughout life. People moving into a fluoridated area after teeth have erupted also benefit.

However, many communities do not have piped water and for geographical and political reasons it has not been possible to fluoridate all water supplies. Consequently, a great deal of research has been carried out to develop alternative methods of supplementing fluoride intake. The aim of this chapter is to discuss this supplementation of fluoride in terms of efficacy and safety. It is outside the scope of this book to discuss the extensive epidemiological investigations, human clinical trials, and animal laboratory studies that have been carried out in relation to fluoride and caries or to cover the physiology of fluoride. The reader is referred to two books on fluoride. One is by Murray, Rugg-Gunn, and Jenkins[5] and the other is by Ekstrand, Fejerskov, and Silverstone.[6]

7.2 CRYSTALLINE STRUCTURE OF ENAMEL[6]

Enamel mineral is crystalline and has a lattice structure characteristic of hydroxyapatite, the smallest repeating unit of which can be expressed by the formula $Ca_{10} (PO_4) (OH)_2$. However, it is not a pure hydroxyapatite since it also has a non-apatite phase (amorphous calcium phosphate or carbonate) and additional ions or molecules are adsorbed on to the large surface area of the apatite crystals. It is important to understand that enamel is essentially a porous structure, allowing ions to diffuse into it. Indeed, the composition of its hydroxyapatite lattice can vary throughout, markedly affecting its structure. This can happen in several different ways:

1. The crystal lattice has the capacity to substitute other ionic species of appropriate size and charge. Thus within the lattice, calcium can be exchanged for radium, strontium, lead, and hydrogen ions while phosphate can be exchanged for carbonate, and hydroxyl for fluoride.
2. Sodium, magnesium, and carbonate can be substituted or adsorbed at the crystal surface.
3. There may be defects present in the internal lattice.
4. It is also possible for part of the lattice to be lost without the whole crystal disintegrating. Similarly, remineralization can occur.

7.2.1 Deposition of fluoride in enamel

There is a great deal of scope to affect the fluoride concentration of enamel since it can be deposited in three stages of enamel development. Low concentrations, reflecting the low levels of fluoride in tissue fluids, are incorporated in the apatite crystals during their formation. After calcification is complete, but before eruption, more fluoride is taken up by the surface enamel which is in contact with the tissue fluids. Finally, after eruption and throughout life, the enamel continues to take up fluoride from its external environment. At this time, the uptake of fluoride will be influenced by the state of the enamel, i.e. whether it is sound or whether acid-etching or caries have made it more porous by preferentially dissolving its interprismatic constituents. Any such increase in porosity facilitates the diffusion and uptake of fluoride by enamel. Enamel from newly erupted teeth also takes up more fluoride than mature enamel.

The fluoride content of intact surface enamel is much higher than the interior enamel but tends to be extremely variable. It varies between primary and permanent teeth, between different individuals living in the same area, between different teeth in the same individual, and even between different surfaces of the same tooth. In carious enamel, white-spot or brown-spot lesions, fluoride levels are raised whereas in areas worn by attrition the levels are low.

7.3 CARIOSTATIC MECHANISMS OF FLUORIDE[5]

Several methods of supplementing fluoride, using many different vehicles containing varying concentrations of fluoride, have been tested over five decades and there is no doubt that such additional fluoride exerts a protective action against dental caries. There is also sufficient evidence to show that fluoride acts in several different ways both before and after tooth eruption:

1. Once teeth have erupted, fluoride inhibits demineralization and pro-
    motes remineralization, thus encouraging repair or arrest of carious
    lesions, delaying lesion progression.
2. Depending on its concentration and pH, fluoride can also exert a bacte-
    ricidal or antienzymatic effect. At the concentration (over 1 per cent F)
    used for topical applications in the dental clinic, fluoride has been
    shown to be toxic to mutans streptococci. Low concentrations (2–10
    ppm F) can inhibit the enzymes involved in acid production and the
    transport and storage of glucose and glucose analogues in oral strepto-
    cocci. It can also interfere with the synthesis of intracellular polysac-
    charides and so restrict the build-up of a reserve supply for acid
    production. Thus the presence of low concentrations of ionic fluoride in
    plaque can reduce the effect of a cariogenic challenge by reducing acid
    production and the consequent fall in pH. In order to be effective, the
    fluoride has to be in ionic form. Although much of the fluoride in
    plaque is a loosely bound fraction, it can be liberated when the pH is
    reduced to 4–5 and so augment the low concentration of ionic fluoride
    (0.9 ppm F) normally present in plaque fluid.
3. Although it is generally accepted that the topical post-eruptive effect of
    fluoride is of prime importance, it may also act on the developing teeth
    before eruption by altering their morphology, making fissures more
    self-cleansing. However, this role of fluoride is still controversial: some
    dismiss any pre-eruptive benefit, while others argue that it is consider-
    able. This is because several factors are involved in the initiation and
    progress of dental caries, and it has been difficult to determine precisely
    which mechanism of action of fluoride predominates.

The majority view on the cariostatic mechanisms of fluoride is as
follows:[7]

1. The predominant effect of fluoride is exerted topically and the pre-
    eruptive effective is minimal.
2. For its effect to last fluoride exposure must be continued after eruption.
3. Fluoride does not appear to have much influence on the initiation of a
    carious lesion, but can greatly retard its rate of progression.
4. It is more important to provide low concentrations of fluoride in the
    environment of the early lesion than to incorporate it into sound
    enamel.
5. Fluoride supplements in the form of tablets or drops have been associ-
    ated with fluorosis.

These statements have implications regarding the appropriate uses of
fluoride, both systemically and topically. If the effect of fluoride on teeth
before they erupt is minimal, it becomes very important to assess the risk of

fluorosis against any small benefit gained by prescribing fluoride tablets or drops for ingestion.

7.4 FLUOROSIS[6]

7.4.1 Signs of fluorosis

The first sign of excessive intake of fluoride during the period of tooth formation is the eruption of teeth with fluorosed or mottled enamel. Its appearance varies from fine white lines in the enamel to chalky, opaque enamel which turns brown or black after eruption. The enamel may even break apart soon after tooth eruption. Fortunately, this most severe form is unusual in the UK. The severity of change depends on the amount of fluoride ingested, its timing, and individual susceptibility due to factors such as body weight.

In order to see the early stages of fluorosis the teeth need to be cleaned and dried and examined in a good light. When fluorosis is mild, enamel merely loses its lustre and, when dried, opaque white flecks or patches can be seen (Fig. 7.1a). It is difficult to distinguish cases of mild fluorosis from other opacities of enamel due to infections in childhood, genetic causes, or trauma. However, such opacities are not usually aesthetically objectionable and it has been suggested that the very early changes may actually enhance the appearance of the teeth.

More obvious mottling or striations (Fig. 7.1b), with or without yellow or brown stains, are apparent in moderate cases of enamel fluorosis and are not acceptable by patients or their parents. When the condition is very severe, pitting occurs and the enamel is so hypoplastic that pieces break off very easily (Fig. 7.1c).

7.4.2 Mechanism of fluorosis

The exact mechanism is not fully understood, but fluoride is thought to affect ameloblast function during both the secretory and the maturation phases, leading to defective mineralization. Fluorosis can be caused by a single high fluoride dose, lower but multiple doses, and by low-level continuous exposure. Consequently, it can be produced by ingestion of fluoride from the drinking water (see Fig. 7.2)[8] and toothpaste as well as by use of dietary fluoride supplements. Although permanent teeth go on developing from birth to adolescence, it is the anterior teeth that are of most concern from an aesthetic viewpoint. Thus the most critical time is from birth to 8 years but the risk is greatest during the first two years of life.[9]

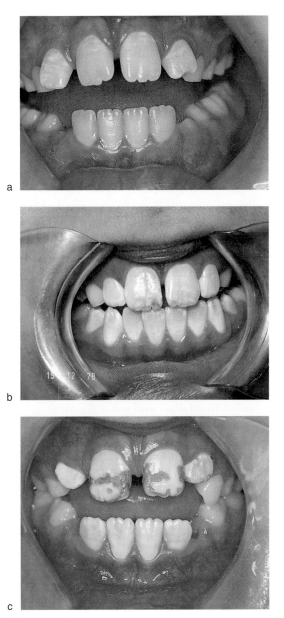

Fig. 7.1. (a) Mild fluorosis. Note white flecks on upper anterior teeth. (b) Moderate fluorosis. Note white striations and yellow-brown discoloration on central incisors. (c) Severe fluorosis. Note loss of enamel.

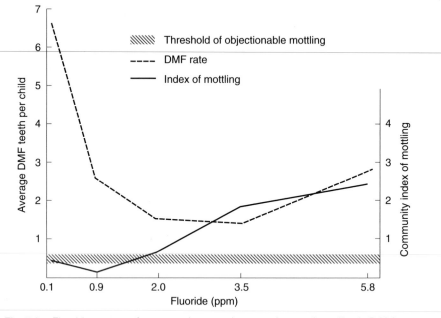

Fig. 7.2. Fluoride content of water: caries experience and enamel mottling in British children aged 12–14 years. (From Forest (1956).[8] Reproduced by courtesy of the Editor, *British Dental Journal*.)

Dietary fluoride supplementation and water fluoridation are not equivalent methods of fluoride exposure. As supplements are generally administered as single doses, either daily or periodically, they produce much higher peaks of fluoride in the plasma than the multiple divided doses received from the water supply. Some believe that this is more likely to produce fluorosis but this has yet to be proven. As early as 1974 Assenden and Peebles[10] reported that the prevalence of mild dental fluorosis in a group of children who had ingested 0.5 mg fluoride from birth to 3 years and 1 mg thereafter was almost twice as high as that of group receiving optimal water fluoridation. As a result of this study the dosage was reduced.

The fluorosis illustrated in Figs 7.1a–c, was caused by excessive fluoride supplementation. The subjects all gave a history of supplemental fluoride drops or tablets at a daily dose of 0.5 mg F from birth to 2 years and 1 mg F thereafter which was the dosage originally recommended before the advent of fluoridated toothpaste. Since these children were also having their teeth brushed with a fluoridated paste twice a day from the age of six to eight months, it is not difficult to see why fluorosis resulted, as their total daily intake would have been in excess of 1.0 mg F.

The cases illustrated in Figs 7.1a–c suggest that there may be a variation in the response of these three children to fluoride. The histories revealed that there was also a variation in their ability to rinse and spit out after brushing. The child with severe fluorosis (Fig. 7.1c) had difficulty rinsing until the age of 8 years. Therefore, in order to avoid fluorosis, it is necessary to restrict the quantity of fluoridated toothpaste used, particularly in children who are also ingesting a fluoride supplement.

In recent years, the amount of fluoride ingested from toothpastes, mouthwashes, and preparations for topical application has increased, and fluoride dosage regimens worldwide have been revised downwards to reduce the risk of fluorosis.

7.5 WHICH FLUORIDE SUPPLEMENT?

Before considering supplementing fluoride, it is relevant to take into account the natural sources of fluoride in food. Seafood and tea are the principal dietary sources of this ion. In fish, it is the skin and bones which contain significant amounts of fluoride. These parts of the fish become edible during canning so that canned fish may contain 9 ppm F. An average infusion of tea, depending on the brand, contains between 1.4 and 4.3 ppm F. Although tea consumption in the UK is high, there is no evidence that this has a beneficial effect on the dental health of the population. This may be because sugar is frequently added to tea.

Fluoride in fish will only be relevant if fish forms a major part of the diet. Similarly, only individuals consuming a very large volume of unsweetened tea might be expected to benefit dentally. Thus, for most people fluoride supplementation from foods is not practical and some other form of fluoride supplement should be considered.

To obtain the maximum benefit from fluoride, its transient presence is required soon after the initial caries attack. Since there is no way of knowing exactly when this is occurring, the aim has to be regular and frequent exposure of the enamel to fluoride to arrest the early lesion. Indeed, there is clinical evidence to suggest that regular use of preparations containing low concentrations of fluoride is more effective than irregular use of agents containing higher concentrations. Furthermore, it has also been shown that when exposure to fluoride is discontinued, its caries-reducing effect gradually wanes. This is entirely logical, because fluoride is affecting the dynamics of lesion formation.

These factors have to be taken into consideration when choosing a fluoride supplement and the regime to be employed. Ultimately, however, the choice must be governed by the dental needs of the individual patient. Since available vehicles for fluoride supplementation contain varying amounts of fluoride it is also necessary to consider the safety of the fluoride preparation chosen in terms of fluorosis and toxicity.

Fluoride is used at home in mouthrinses and toothpaste or applied in the dental surgery in the form of varnishes, topical solutions, gels, or prophylaxis pastes. If some of these preparations are accidentally swallowed during the period of tooth formation there is a potential for fluorosis. Fluoride may also affect developing enamel, if ingested as fluoridated water, sodium fluoride tablets or drops or fluoridated salt.

7.5.1 Fluoride in drinking water

There is no doubt that adding fluoride to the drinking water is the most effective, safest, and cheapest way of preventing caries. It works both before and after the teeth erupt, and has the added advantage that no conscious cooperation on the part of the individual is required. Indeed, it satisfies the criteria for the ideal fluoride supplement—a low, safe concentration used regularly and frequently to delay lesion progression. However, optimally fluoridated water is available to only 10 per cent of the UK population. A recent report of the national survey of children's dental health[11] reveals major differences in caries incidence across the UK: the prevalence in Scotland and Northern Ireland is much higher than in England, particularly in socially deprived sections of population. These high-risk communities in particular would benefit most from fluoridation. Unfortunately, until this comes about we have to choose from alternative methods of supplementing the natural supply of fluoride.

7.6 DIETARY FLUORIDE SUPPLEMENTS

7.6.1 Fluoride tablets

Dosage regimes vary considerably between countries, which has caused some concern among manufacturers in Europe because of the European labelling regulations. If multi-language instructions are included with the containers, each will present different recommended levels, confusing the public. An international seminar of European experts in 1993 agreed that dietary fluoride supplements need only be taken by individuals at high risk of dental caries—i.e. medically compromised children and those with caries or increased susceptibility. For over-the-counter sales, the dose level advised is 0.5 mg from the age of 3 years in places where the fluoride content of the water supply is deficient. However, the group recognized that individual children might have different needs and that a dentist should feel free to prescribe outside this rigid regimen in the interests of each patient.

Recommended fluoride dosages

The authors strongly recommend adopting a regimen in line with that suggested for the rest of Europe. There is little point in prescribing supplements for children who have never experienced caries, because they are very unlikely to continue the regimen. Those who do continue to use supplements are likely to be children of dentally conscious, middle-class parents who will also brush their children's teeth regularly, resulting in ingestion of additional fluoride from the dentifrice, and running a greater risk of their children developing fluorosis. The reviews by Szpunar and Burt[7] and Riordan[9] provide compelling evidence of the risk of fluorosis from tablets, particularly if they are given to children as young as six months of age. It is generally more appropriate to tackle caries control in the pre-school child by concentrating on dietary advice and combining this with an application of fluoride varnish in the surgery at a later stage for the high-risk patient.

Dietary fluoride supplements need only ever be prescribed for children at high risk of dental caries—medically compromised children and those already suffering from caries—*providing* the water supply contains less than 0.3 ppm fluoride. The regime recommended is as follows:

1. The recommended dose level for over-the-counter preparations is 0.5 mg F daily from the age of 3 years.
2. When susceptibility is so great that caries is diagnosed before the age of 3 years, the individual child may be prescribed 0.25 mg F daily until the age of 3 years. This should be increased to 0.5mg F daily after 3 years.
3. Whenever possible, fluoride tablets should be allowed to dissolve slowly in the mouth to produce a topical effect and, if practical, the dose should be split and administered on two occasions each day. Ideally, children should take the tablets at a different time from toothbrushing because they will inevitably swallow some toothpaste, which will increase the plasma fluoride level. By staggering the time, an additional topical effect will be provided.
4. Young children should always be supervised when brushing; a low-fluoride paste should be used and the amount placed on the brush should be limited to the size of a small pea. This is imperative if the dietary fluoride supplements are being used.
5. Supplements should not be used if the water is fluoridated or if it contains more than 0.3 ppm fluoride. The fluoride content of any bottled

water used should be checked: those marketed in the UK contain between 0.1 and 0.8 ppm fluoride.[12]

7.6.2 Fluoridated salt

Hungary, Switzerland, France, and Germany have used fluoridated salt as an alternative to water fluoridation with considerable success. Careful studies have also been carried out in Columbia and Spain. The current concentration is 250 mg F/kg. However, the actual amount of fluoride taken in by individuals will vary with the amount of salt a person eats, and may be a problem.

7.6.3 Pre-natally administered fluoride

The benefit from pre-natal supplementation of fluoride is uncertain. It has been shown that some fluoride ingested by the pregnant woman passes through the placenta to the fetus. However, the concentration of fluoride in foetal tissues is low and does not seem to be linearly related to the fluoride intake by the mother. In the light of present knowledge, and the extremely small benefit that could be gained, there is no justification for the administration of fluoride tablets during pregnancy.

7.7 FLUORIDE PREPARATIONS FOR TOPICAL APPLICATION

A number of preparations are available for topical application of fluoride. These fall into two categories:

- frequent-use, low-concentration preparations (toothpastes and mouthrinses)
- periodic-use, high-concentration preparations (sodium fluoride varnishes, acidulated phosphate fluoride and stannous fluoride gels, and prophylaxis pastes).

7.7.1 Toothpastes

The use of fluoride toothpastes has contributed greatly to the decline of caries in industrial countries. Regular use of fluoride toothpastes is the most practical way of keeping fluoride concentrations at the plaque–enamel interface high, and its use should be recommended for all patients.

The vast majority of toothpastes currently contain sodium fluoride, sodium monofluorophosphate, or a mixture of both and fluoride concentrations range from 525 to 1450 ppm F. Toothpaste formulation is complex and numerous clinical trials have been undertaken showing the superiority of one product or another.[5] However, these studies are often not comparable and differences are, at best, marginal. Consequently, it is difficult, if not impossible to choose a brand to recommend, bearing in mind that all the main brands are effective.

The following guidelines should be followed to reduce the risk of fluorosis:

1. *Pre-school children:* Children under the age of 5 years cannot rinse adequately and they may ingest more than 0.5 mg fluoride daily from two brushings of toothpaste containing between 1000 and 1450 ppm F because a brush full of a 1000 ppm F paste contains about 1 mg fluoride. These very young children should use a low-fluoride toothpaste (500 to 600 ppm F), in the following way:

- only a small pea-sized amount of paste should be applied to the child-size toothbrush
- parents should apply the paste to the brush and brush their children's teeth until the child can do it properly
- children should be encouraged to spit the paste out after brushing.

These guidelines assume even greater importance when dietary fluoride supplements are given.

2. *Children over the age of 8 years:* For children over the age of 8 years who would be outside the window of vulnerability to fluorosis of the anterior teeth, it is safe to use the 'family' toothpaste containing high levels of fluoride. However, if dietary fluoride supplements are prescribed for a high-risk child, it is safer for this child to use a low-fluoride paste if they are likely to brush without supervision.

3. *Adults:* It is always worth checking that adults are using a toothpaste containing fluoride: high-risk patients sometimes select a toothpaste for sensitive teeth which does not contain fluoride. The patient should be encouraged to change to a comparable fluoride-containing product.

7.7.2 Mouthrinses

The daily, weekly, or fortnightly use of a fluoride mouthrinse is a valuable anticaries measure in high-risk patients who live in areas where the water supply is low in fluoride. The fluoride concentration advocated in the mouthrinse depends on how frequently it is used. Individuals should rinse for 1 minute with 10 ml of a sodium fluoride solution at a concentration of

0.05 per cent sodium fluoride if used once daily or at 0.2 per cent if used at weekly or fortnightly intervals.

Daily rinsing is marginally more effective than weekly or fortnightly rinsing. Moreover, because of the lower fluoride concentration, daily rinsing is safer for children, provided that they are over 6 years old and can rinse adequately. For adults, choice should depend on patient cooperation. It is easy to forget to rinse weekly or fortnightly, but daily rinsing soon becomes habitual.

Many fluoride rinses are available for sale over the counter in chemist shops and supermarkets. These products contain alcohol to stabilize the preparation and give it an astringent taste. The alcohol content can be as low as 4 per cent (this would be equivalent to some beers) or as high as 27 per cent. It is suggested that a mouthwash with a low alcohol content is chosen for children and patients with dry mouths who may find a high-alcohol mouthwash too astringent and potentially damaging to the oral mucosa. Where the alcohol content of the mouthwash is not stated on the bottle, the manufacturer should be contacted. There are some products on the market which are water based. One of these is sold as a concentrated solution to be diluted with water by the patient. The resulting solution is tasteless, has a neutral pH and contains no alcohol. The disadvantages are that it demands further patient compliance and that the concentrated solution would be hazardous if swallowed by a child.

Indications for use of mouthrinses

The following patients should be encouraged to use mouthrinses:

1. caries-prone children over the age of 6 years provided they can rinse and spit adequately;
2. patients with orthodontic appliances;
3. caries-prone adults, including those whose salivary flow rate has been reduced by drugs, disease, or radiotherapy;
4. adults with exposed root surfaces may also benefit.

A dietary history should always be obtained (see section 6.6.1). Dietary advice, as well as oral hygiene instruction, should always precede a prescription for fluoride.

Contraindications for use of mouthrinses

Mouthrinses should not be used by children under 6 years of age who are not capable of rinsing adequately. They are also unnecessary when fluoride tablets are being taken and allowed to dissolve slowly in the mouth.

7.7.3 Periodic use, high-concentration preparations

When dental apatite is exposed to preparations containing high concentrations of fluoride the major reaction product is calcium fluoride (CaF_2). The slow dissolution and hence prolonged retention of CaF_2, particularly in the early carious lesion, is the key mechanism of the caries-reducing effect of concentrated topical fluoride.

Preparations come in various forms:

1. sodium fluoride varnishes which are painted on in the surgery with a very small brush;
2. APF gels which are swabbed on to the tooth surface or applied in closely fitting trays;
3. stannous fluoride gels which are applied at home with a toothbrush;
4. prophylaxis pastes containing fluoride, which are applied in the surgery with a rubber cup.

The agents available, together with their respective fluoride concentrations and the amount of fluoride per ml, are listed in Table 7.1.

These agents, except for stannous fluoride gels and prophylaxis pastes, have been shown to be equally effective in controlled clinical trials. The choice of agent therefore depends on cost, ease of application, and safety. Fluoride varnish is currently the agent of choice in the UK and Europe because it is easy to apply safely and requires minimal cooperation from the patient. APF (acidulated phosphate fluoride) gels are now rarely used in the UK, but they are still used in the USA and Canada and so are also discussed below.

Sodium fluoride varnish

Duraphat, the product currently available in the UK, contains sodium fluoride in an alcoholic solution of natural varnishes. It is ideally applied on clean dry teeth with a brush but it is water tolerant and will cling onto teeth even if moisture is present. Consequently, it is easier to apply than the

Table 7.1 Topical fluoride agents containing high concentrations of fluoride

Agents available	Concentration	mg F/ml
Sodium fluoride varnish	2.26% F	22
APF gel	1.23% F	12
Stannous fluoride gel	0.4% SnF_2	1
Prophylaxis paste	0.64–1.2% F	1

other fluoride agents. The fluoride concentration is high (22 mg/ml), but the total amount of fluoride ingested is less than after gel application because only a small quantity needs to be applied. It has the added advantage that it need only be applied to vulnerable surfaces and not to the whole dentition.

Indications: Application of sodium fluoride varnish is indicated for the following groups of patients:

1. Caries-prone adults who cannot or will not use a fluoride mouthrinse.
2. Patients with removable orthodontic appliances and partial dentures (biannual applications).
3. Children over 6 years and adults exposed to a greater cariogenic challenge because their dietary habits have changed since their last visit due to illness, change of school, or occupation.
4. Localized application to initial carious lesions where the clinician hopes to arrest lesion progression and to protect vulnerable exposed root surfaces.
5. In exceptional cases, when it is difficult to control caries in children under 6 years, a small quantity of varnish may be carefully painted on each lesion followed by gentle washing with water.

Contraindications: Home use of fluoride varnish is contraindicated for patients for safety reasons. It is also generally contraindicated in the surgery for children under the age of 6 years.

APF gel

When the gel is applied in a tray, between 19 and 75 per cent of the gel can be swallowed depending on whether a saliva ejector is used. If the gel is swallowed in sufficient quantity it is very toxic (Table 7.2), so a very careful application technique must be employed. Its use is not generally recommended in the UK. However, if it is used the following guidelines should be observed.

1. Trays should not be used for applying gels in children under 16 years of age; it is safer to swab the fluoride gel only on selected teeth.
2. The dental chair should be upright and the patient should lean forward.
3. The tray must be closely fitting and only a thin ribbon of gel, not more than 2 ml per tray should be applied.
4. A saliva ejector must be used.
5. Patients should be instructed to spit out thoroughly immediately following application and suction should be used to evacuate the mouth.

Table 7.2   Toxicity of fluoride preparations, calculated for a 5-year-old child weighing 20 kg

		Sublethal acute poisoning dose	Potentially lethal poisoning dose
APF gel (1.23% F)		1.7 ml (1/3 rd teaspoon)	8 ml = 1.5 teaspoons
Sodium fluoride varnish (2.26% F)		0.9 ml (1/5th teaspoon)	4 ml = 4/5th teaspoon
Stannous fluoride gel (0.4% SnF$_2$)		20 ml (4 teaspoons)	100 ml = 1 cup
Rinse (0.2% NaF)		22 ml (1/5th cup)	105 ml = 1 cup
Rinse (0.05% NaF)		88 ml (4/5th cup)	420 ml = 4 cups
Rinse concentrate (2.0% NaF)		2.2 ml (1/2 teaspoon)	10 ml = 2 teaspoons
Tablets:	0.5 mg F	40 tablets	200 tablets
	1.0 mg F	20 tablets	100 tablets
Toothpaste:*	500 ppm	66 ml	200 ml
	1000 ppm	33 ml	100 ml
	1500 ppm	22 ml	66 ml

* Toothpaste tubes generally contain 50, 100, or 125 ml.

Stannous fluoride gel

These gels contain 0.4 per cent stannous fluoride and are applied with a toothbrush by the patient following normal toothbrushing and rinsing last thing at night. No rinsing, eating, or drinking is allowed after expectoration of excess gel.

The cariostatic effect of this preparation has not been demonstrated in controlled clinical trials but there are reports that susceptibility to caries in orthodontic and post-irradiation patients is reduced. Using a fluoride toothpaste with an equivalent fluoride concentration (1000 ppm) in the same way (i.e. without rinsing) may well have the same effect. Mild staining of teeth due to the tin content has limited the use of these gels in many countries.

Contraindications: Stannous fluoride gel should not be used in children under 6 years and those who are taking dietary fluoride supplements. Patients with reduced salivary flow may also experience mucosal irritation because it is recommended that the patient does not rinse after brushing with the gel.

Prophylaxis pastes

These pastes are not recommended as agents to supplement fluoride because the use of any abrasive agent results in the loss of surface enamel which contains a high concentration of fluoride. Thus the net loss of fluoride may be equal to, or greater than, the net gain. Unless staining is severe, a fluoride-containing toothpaste can effectively be used for prophylaxis. If a prophylaxis paste is to be used, one which contains fluoride and which is only mildly abrasive should be chosen.

Topical fluoride application in optimally fluoridated areas

Results of studies on the value of topically applied fluorides for children in such areas are not clear cut. Nevertheless, the highly susceptible individual should be given professional applications of a topical fluoride preparation or asked to use a fluoride mouthrinse. It is important, however, to exclude children under the age of 6 years.

7.8 TOXICITY

Anyone recommending the use of fluoride-containing dental preparations should be aware of the fluoride content and the potential hazards. Information on the toxicity of fluoride in humans is gathered from recorded cases of deliberate or accidental overdosage. The acute lethal dose is approximately 15 mg/kg body weight, although as little as 5 mg/kg may kill some children.[6] A dose of 5 mg/kg should trigger immediate emergency treatment. As little as 1 mg/kg can produce sublethal toxic effects.

The exact mechanism by which fluoride produces its toxic effect is not known. Symptoms of sublethal poisoning are salivation, nausea and vomiting. The symptoms usually appear within an hour of ingestion and, if overdosage occurs as a result of topical fluoride application, may not be manifest until the patient has left the surgery. Death from respiratory or cardiac failure occurs within 24 hours of a lethal dose.

A small quantity of fluoride (less than 5 mg/kg body weight) is neutralized by drinking a large volume of milk. However, if more than 5 mg/kg have been ingested or if there is any doubt about the exact quantity consumed, the child should be taken to hospital and given gastric lavage. Speed is of the utmost importance because fluoride is very rapidly absorbed.

Table 7.2 lists some of the fluoride agents in use, the amount required to produce early toxic effects and the potential lethal dose—all in relation to the average 5-year-old weighing about 20 kg (44 lb). These values would be considerably lower for the average 2-year-old. It is apparent that for a 5-year-old, as far as APF gels are concerned, as little as one-third of a teaspoonful can produce toxic effects and one and a half teaspoonfuls can be lethal. Sodium fluoride varnish is even more concentrated so that as little as four-fifths of a teaspoonful is dangerous for the young child.

Consequently, if fluoride varnish is used in exceptional cases in pre-school children, extreme care must be exercised. For children over the age of 6 years, a fluoride varnish should be chosen because, although the fluoride concentration is high, only a small quantity is applied and, unlike gels in trays, a safe technique requires minimal cooperation from a child.

Although no cases of acute toxicity due to ingestion of toothpaste have ever been reported, a 5-year-old could be severely poisoned by consuming about two-thirds of a 100 ml tube of 1500 ppm fluoride paste; a 1-year-old would need to consume only half this amount. Fluoride toothpaste should therefore be kept out of the reach of young children.

7.9 SUMMARY

1. Fluoride acts by retarding the progression of caries rather than by preventing its initiation.
2. It is more important to provide low concentrations of fluoride in the environment of the early lesion than to incorporate it into the enamel.
3. The main effect of fluoride is exerted topically and the pre-eruptive effect is minimal.
4. Dietary fluoride supplements should be considered only for patients at high risk of caries. The revised tablet regimen recommended should be adopted because of the risk of fluorosis.
5. Dietary fluoride supplementation is contraindicated when the water supply is optimally fluoridated or contains more than 0.3 ppm fluoride.
6. Topical fluoride preparations should be applied carefully because of their potential toxic effects. Fluoride varnish is the topical agent of choice, especially for high-risk patients whose compliance with home regimes, such as fluoride rinses, may be a problem.
7. Parents should always supervise young children's use of toothpaste.
8. Dental products for home use, including toothpaste, should be kept out of the reach of young children.
9. The use of fluorides in dental practice should always be combined with dietary advice and oral hygiene instruction and should be tailored to the needs of the individual patient.

REFERENCES

1. McKay, F.S. (1916). An investigation into mottled teeth (1). *Dental Cosmos.*, **58**, 477–84.
2. Churchill, H.V. (1931). The occurrence of fluorides in some waters of the United States. *J. Dent. Res.*, **12**, 141–8.

3. Ainsworth, N.J. (1933). Mottled teeth. *Br. Dent. J.*, **55,** 233–50.

4. Dean, H.T., Arnold, F.A., and Evolve, E. (1942). Domestic water and dental caries V, additional studies of the relation of fluoride domestic waters to dental caries experience in 4,425 white children aged 12–14 years, of 13 cities in 4 States. *Public Health Rep.*, **57**, 1155–79.

5. Murray, J.J., Rugg–Gunn, A., and Jenkins, G.N. (1991). *Fluorides in caries prevention*, (3rd edn). Butterworth-Heinemann, Oxford.

6. Ekstrand, J., Fejerskov, O., and Silverstone, L.M. (1988). *Fluoride in dentistry.* Munksgaard, Copenhagen.

7. Szpunar, S.M. and Burt, B.A. (1992). Evaluation of appropriate use of dietary fluoride supplements in the U.S. *Community Dent. Oral Epidemiol.*, **20**, 148–54.

8. Forest, J.R. (1956). Caries experience and enamel defects in areas with different levels of fluoride in the drinking water. *Br. Dent. J.*, **100**, 195–200.

9. Riordan, P.J. (1993). Fluoride supplements in caries prevention: a literature review and proposal for a new dosage schedule. *J. Public Health Dent.*, **53**, 174–89.

10. Assenden, R. and Peebles, T.C. (1974). Effects of fluoride supplementation from birth on human deciduous and permanent teeth. *Arch. Oral Biol.*, **19**, 321–6.

11. Downer, M.C. (1995). The 1993 National Survey of children's dental health. *Br. Dent. J.*, **178**, 407–12.

12. Toumba, K.J., Levy, S., and Curzon, M.E.J. (1994). The fluoride content of bottled drinking waters. *Br. Dent. J.*, **176**, 266–8.

8

Prevention of caries by plaque control

8.1 INTRODUCTION[1]

Caries is a process in which bacterial plaque interacts with the diet and the resistance of the host. Without plaque no caries would be initiated. Thus plaque control is of fundamental importance in the management of the carious process.

In the past there has been much argument about which bacteria are cariogenic. The *non-specific plaque hypothesis* suggests that all plaque is potentially cariogenic. This would imply that daily, mechanical plaque removal is important in the management of the carious process. The *specific plaque hypothesis*, on the other hand, proposes that plaque is not always cariogenic and that only certain plaques, colonized by specific microorganisms, are responsible for dental decay. This would imply that targeting of specific organisms, such as mutans streptococci, might control the carious process. This approach is the rationale behind considering the use of topical antimicrobials such as chlorhexidine, in the management of dental caries.

In recent years the *ecological plaque hypothesis* has been proposed and this appears to combine the two previous approaches. The argument behind the ecological plaque hypothesis can be summarized as follows:

1. Cariogenic bacteria are found naturally in dental plaque.
2. At neutral pH these organisms are a small proportion of the total plaque community.
3. With a conventional diet, the processes of de- and remineralization are in equilibrium and the carious process does not progress.
4. If the frequency of carbohydrate intake increases, plaque spends more time at an acid pH.
5. This low pH favours the proliferation of mutans streptococci and lactobacilli and tips the balance towards demineralization.
6. Now greater numbers of mutans streptococci and lactobacilli in plaque produce acid at faster rates, enhancing demineralization.

This hypothesis explains the lack of total specificity in the microbial aetiology of dental caries. It explains the pattern of bacterial succession and shows why both the approach of total plaque removal and chemical targeting of specific microorganisms may have a role to play in the management of dental caries.

The following two methods of plaque control will now be discussed in detail:

1. mechanical removal of plaque;
2. chemical methods to inhibit plaque formation or to eliminate specific bacteria and their products within plaque.

8.2 MECHANICAL REMOVAL OF PLAQUE

8.2.1 Seeing plaque: disclosing agents and mirrors

In order to learn how to remove plaque effectively it is helpful for the patient to see where it is present. Since plaque is translucent and has a colour similar to teeth, it must be stained in order to be seen clearly (see Figs. 1.4a,b, p. 6). Liquids, tablets, and capsules containing erythrosin or vegetable dyes are used to stain plaque and are called 'disclosing agents'. Once a patient has been taught to identify plaque, the disclosing agent should be applied after toothbrushing so that areas where oral hygiene is inadequate can be seen easily. However, this will only be possible if the bathroom mirror used at home by the patient is well illuminated and a mouth mirror is also used. An inexpensive magnifying shaving mirror together with a disposable mouth mirror (Fig. 8.1) are invaluable aids for effective oral hygiene. When adequate lighting is a problem a mirror–light combination is a good solution.

8.2.2 Toothbrushes

Toothbrushes vary widely in shape and size of the head, the material, texture, and arrangement of filaments as well as in the size and shape of the handles. However, at present nearly all toothbrushes available are multitufted with nylon filaments. Attempts have been made to establish the relative importance of the other variables in design but the results have been inconclusive. This is not surprising, since the efficiency of a toothbrush in removing plaque is, for the most part, dependent on the care the subject exercises and to a very minor degree on the type of brush and method of brushing. Any toothbrush which allows a particular patient to reach all tooth surfaces easily and comfortably is acceptable, although a medium brush with a small head is generally recommended. It is particularly important that brushes are replaced regularly, at least every three months or sooner if the bristles become permanently bent. A brush which shows such signs of wear cannot clean effectively. Although there is considerable variation in manual dexterity, most healthy individuals can be taught to clean

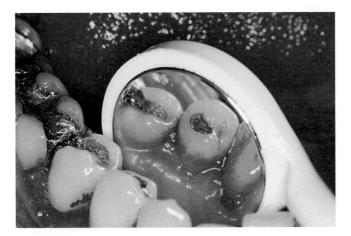

Fig. 8.1. A disposable mouth mirror allows the patient to see plaque on lingual and interproximal areas.

their teeth effectively, provided they are sufficiently motivated. However, for the physically handicapped, where manual dexterity is limited, an electric toothbrush is very helpful.

8.2.3 Methods of toothbrushing

Various methods of toothbrushing have been advocated and classified according to the type of motion performed by the brush:

1. The 'scrub' method is performed by using a *horizontal* scrubbing motion and is usually recommended for children.
2. In the 'Charters' and 'Bass' methods a *vibratory* motion is used.

In reality it does not matter exactly how a toothbrush is used as long as plaque is removed effectively without trauma to the gingival tissues. Disclosing agents will show areas where plaque removal is ineffective. The patient should now be asked to clean these areas as they would normally. Where plaque still persists the professional should teach effective oral hygiene. The recommended method will depend upon the dexterity of the individual patient as well as configuration of the teeth. The vibratory Charters and Bass techniques are most useful and will be described in detail.

The Charters method (Fig. 8.2)

The brush is held with the bristles *pointing towards the occlusal* plane and then applied to the teeth at an angle of 45° to this plane. The brush is pressed so that the bristles are flexed and the tips forced between the teeth.

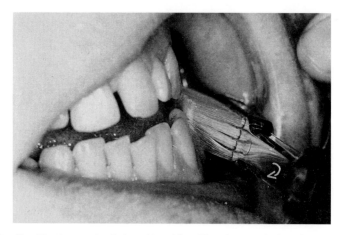

Fig. 8.2.   The Charters method of toothbrushing. Note the angulation of the bristles against the tooth surface.

It is then vibrated by a rotary movement of the handle, keeping the tips of the bristles in position. This method of brushing is advocated in patients with open interdental spaces because it facilitates the penetration of the brush filaments.

The Bass method (Fig. 8.3)

The brush is held so that the bristles are directed *apically* and then placed against the gingival margin at an angle of 45° to the long axis of the tooth. The brush is then vibrated in an anterior–posterior direction. In order to clean the lingual surfaces of the upper and lower anterior teeth the brush has to be turned into a vertical position, using the bristles at the 'toe' of the brush to obtain proper access to the gingival area of the teeth.

The Bass method is effective in removing plaque adjacent to and directly below the gingival margin. Since the bristles of the brush are directed towards the gingival tissues and may be potentially damaging a hard brush must not be used with this method.

Some patients will pick up a new cleaning technique easily while others find it difficult. It is sometimes helpful to guide the patient's hand so that they can feel the motion required.

8.2.4 Interdental cleaning

Approximal surfaces and areas where teeth are malaligned cannot be reached with an ordinary toothbrush. Consequently, additional aids such as

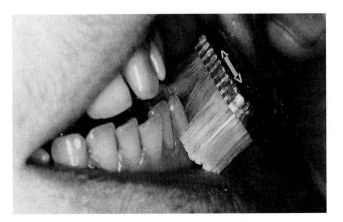

Fig. 8.3. The Bass method of toothbrushing. Note the angulation of the bristles against the tooth surface and the direction of the vibratory motion.

dental floss or tape, woodsticks, single-tufted brushes, or interdental brushes may be required for these areas. Choice will depend on the shape of the interdental area and the dexterity of the individual.

Dental floss or tape

In a young and healthy mouth where the interdental papillae fill the interdental spaces, the use of dental floss or tape is the method of choice for interproximal cleaning. No differences have been found in cleansing potential between waxed and unwaxed floss although unwaxed floss tends to fray more readily.

It is necessary to teach the patient the correct technique for applying floss otherwise damage to the gingival tissues is likely. The correct technique is illustrated in Figs. 8.4 and 8.5. The fingers holding the floss should not be more than half an inch apart. The floss should be guided slowly through the contact point and then wrapped around the interproximal surface of each tooth in turn. A sawing motion along the surface is then used to remove plaque. The index fingers of both hands are usually used to control the floss when the lower teeth are cleaned (Fig. 8.4). For the upper teeth it is recommended that the index finger of one hand and the thumb of the other hand are used (Fig. 8.5). A clean section of floss should be used for each interproximal space. Patients who are sufficiently motivated can usually learn to floss adequately, although some patients take longer to grasp the technique. In such patients patent floss holders may be helpful (see Fig. 8.6).

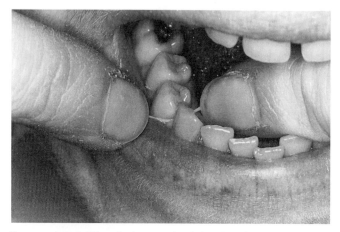

Fig. 8.4.   The use of dental floss for interproximal cleaning of the lower teeth. Two index fingers are used to control the floss.

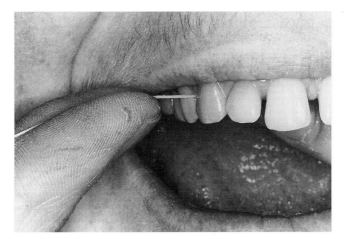

Fig. 8.5. The use of dental floss for interproximal cleaning of the upper teeth. The floss is controlled by the index finger of one hand and the thumb of the other.

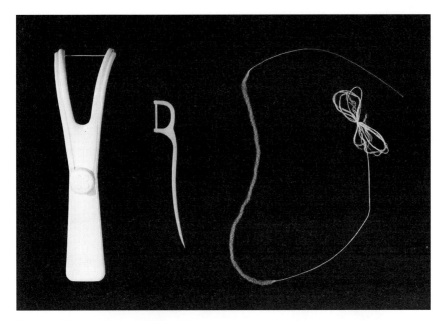

Fig. 8.6. Floss holders and 'Super' floss.

'Super' floss (see also Fig. 8.6) is specially designed to clean under bridge-work. A section of the floss, about 12 cm long, is thickened with a foamlike material and when threaded under a bridge is very effective in removing plaque (Fig. 8.7).

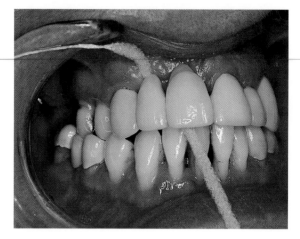

Fig. 8.7. The use of 'Super' floss to remove plaque under a bridge.

Woodsticks

When there is recession of the interdental papillae and consequently inter-dental spaces are present, woodsticks can be used for interpromixal clean-ing instead of dental floss.

Woodsticks are made of soft wood and are triangular in shape so that they fit the interdental space. The base of the wedge is applied to the gingi-val border of the interdental area with the tip pointing towards the occlusal plane (Fig. 8.8). The interproximal surfaces are then cleaned by moving the woodstick in and out, applying pressure on each side of the embrasure

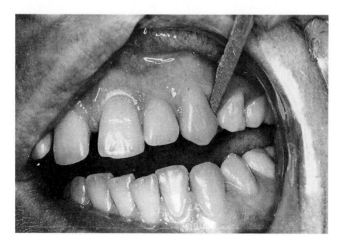

Fig. 8.8. The use of a woodstick for cleaning an interdental area.

in turn. In order to prevent the use of excessive force and to steady the fingers holding the stick, the cheek or chin should be used as a finger rest.

Interdental brushes

When there are wide interdental spaces present, an interdental brush is ideal for the removal of interdental plaque (Fig. 8.9). It is also a useful aid for cleaning around bridges. This brush is shaped like a miniature bottle brush and is available in different sizes (see Fig. 8.10). The smaller brushes

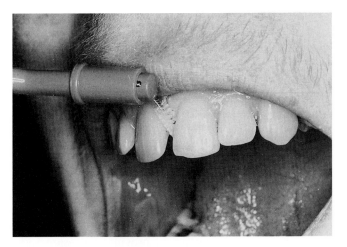

Fig. 8.9. The use of an interdental brush.

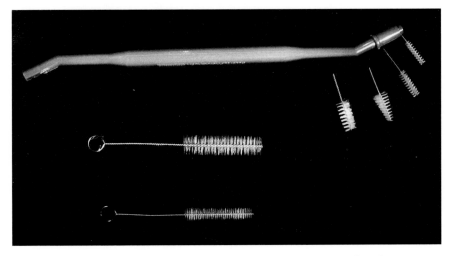

Fig. 8.10. Interdental brushes in various sizes for use with and without a handle.

are usually inserted into handles to make them easier to manipulate. It is important to select the correct size of brush to fit the particular interdental space to be cleaned. It is also important to 'see the patient in action' to be sure they are using it correctly.

Single-tufted brushes

It is often difficult to reach the distal surfaces of posterior teeth or areas where teeth are malaligned. A single-tufted brush (Fig. 8.11) is a very useful additional aid for cleaning these areas.

8.2.5 Dentifrices

In the past dentifrices were used in conjunction with a toothbrush solely for cosmetic and social reasons. However, in the last 30 years fluorides, antibiotics, ammonium compounds, enzyme inhibitors, and bicarbonate have been added in attempts to inhibit dental caries. Of all these agents only fluoride has stood up to clinical testing for safety and efficacy in caries prevention. It is also becoming increasingly common for manufacturers to add other therapeutic or preventive agents to reduce gingivitis and calculus formation. A few toothpastes also contain desensitizing agents. Although the line between the cosmetic and therapeutic actions is not drawn easily, most dentifrices currently on sale have similar objectives. They clean and polish the accessible surfaces of the teeth and provide a pleasant sensation and

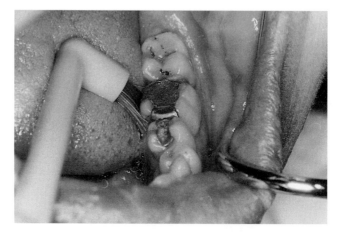

Fig. 8.11. The use of a single-tufted brush for cleaning the lingual surface of a lower molar.

odour to the oral cavity. They also act as a vehicle for applying fluoride to tooth structure.

Composition of dentifrices

Most dentifrices are produced in paste form and have a similar basic formulation. A few powder dentifrices are available containing abrasives, detergents, flavouring, colouring agents, and sweeteners. Toothpastes contain all these agents as well as binding agents, humectants, preservatives, and water (see Table 8.1). Most toothpastes in the UK and the USA also contain fluoride. Many pastes also contain other therapeutic or preventive agents.

The functions of the constituents of toothpaste are as follows:

Cleaning and polishing agents (30–40 per cent): These abrasive agents are the major constituents of toothpastes and may consist of one of the following materials:

- silica
- calcium carbonate
- dicalcium phosphate
- sodium metaphosphate
- hydrated alumina
- zirconium silicate
- calcium pyrophosphate.

Table 8.1 Composition of toothpaste

Cleaning and polishing agents
Detergents
Binding agents
Humectants
Flavouring and sweetening agents
Preservatives
Colouring agents
Therapeutic agents:
    Fluorides
    Desensitizing agents
    Antiplaque agents:
        Triclosan
        Sanguinarine
        Amyloglucosidase and glucose oxidase
    Anticalculus agents
    Bicarbonate
    Xylitol

There is considerable variation in the inherent abrasivity of toothpastes depending upon which abrasive system is used. However, the hardness of the toothbrush and the force used will also affect the actual abrasion experienced. All dentifrices sold in the UK must not exceed a specified level of abrasivity set by the British Standards Institute. In practice, most dentifrices will remove plaque and pellicle without removing significant amounts of enamel. However, if a hard brush is used with force, particularly on exposed root surfaces, abrasion can cause serious loss of dental tissue.

Detergents (1–2 per cent): The purpose of these agents is to facilitate the distribution of the paste in the mouth by lowering the surface tension and helping to loosen plaque and other debris from the tooth surface. They also contribute to the foaming action of toothpastes. The detergents commonly used are sodium lauryl sulphate and sodium N-lauryl sarcosinate.

Binding agents (1–5 per cent): Alginates, gums, or cellulose derivatives such as carboxymethyl cellulose and hydroxyethyl cellulose are used to prevent separation of the solid and liquid ingredients during storage.

Humectants (10–30 per cent): These agents are used to retain moisture and prevent hardening of the paste on exposure to air. Glycerol, sorbitol, and propylene glycol are commonly used.

Flavouring and sweetening agents (1–5 per cent): The taste of a toothpaste is one of its most important selling points. In order to mask the less pleasant taste of some of the other ingredients, flavouring agents such as aromatic oils (peppermint, spearmint, cinnamon, wintergreen) and menthol are added. The glycerol and sorbitol, used as humectants, sweeten the paste. In addition, saccharin may also be used.

Preservatives (0.05–0.5 per cent): Alcohols, benzoates, formaldehyde, and dichlorinated phenols are added to the toothpaste in order to prevent bacterial growth on the organic binders and humectants.

Colouring agents are added to make the product look attractive.

Therapeutic and preventive agents: Many toothpastes now contain therapeutic or preventive agents for specific problems. In order to be effective it is important that these agents do not react with the other constituents of the paste.

   1. *Fluorides.* The caries-reducing effect of toothpaste containing fluoride is in the region of 15–30 per cent. Most of the toothpastes available in the UK contain fluoride as sodium monofluorophosphate or sodium fluoride, separately or together, and fluoride concentrations range from 525 to 1450

ppm F (see Chapter 7). Clinical trials of dentifrices containing fluoride are reviewed elsewhere.[2]

2. *Desensitizing agents.* Toothpastes formulated to alleviate sensitivity of exposed dentine contain one of the following agents: strontium chloride, strontium acetate, formaldehyde, potassium nitrate and chloride, and sodium citrate.

3. *Antiplaque agents.* Several toothpastes contain *triclosan*, an antibacterial agent which is non-ionic (i.e. it has no charge). Unlike other proven cationic (positive charge) plaque inhibiting agents like chlorhexidine, triclosan does not react with the detergents in the dentifrice. However, because it is non-ionic its retention in the mouth is poor but this has been enhanced by combining it with zinc citrate or a copolymer. Such triclosan-containing toothpastes have been shown to reduce plaque formation and gingivitis to some extent. However, the cariostatic effect is not yet adequately proven.

Sanguinarine is a plant alkaloid extract which has been incorporated in a toothpaste because of its antibacterial properties. However, the toothpaste has only been shown to be of some clinical value if it is used in conjunction with a sanguinarine mouthwash.

An oxygenating system using the enzymes *amyloglucosidase* and *glucose oxidase* has been added to a toothpaste to stimulate salivary peroxidase. Theoretically, this, in turn, increases production of hypothiocyanite which has antibacterial properties. However, studies assessing the plaque-inhibiting effects of toothpastes containing the enzymes have produced conflicting results.

4. *Anticalculus agents.* Several different agents have been added to reduce the formation of *supragingival* calculus. These include pyrophosphates, diphosphonates, zinc salts, and Gantrez acid which is a co-polymer of methyl ether and maleic anhydride. Calculus reductions reported for the various systems range between 10 and 50 per cent.

5. *Bicarbonate.* Bicarbonate has recently been added to toothpaste. The rationale for its inclusion is that it is alkaline and may therefore reduce the acidity of dental plaque. This would create a hostile environment for the growth of aciduric bacteria such as mutans streptococci and lactobacilli. There are no reported clinical trials of these formulations in relation to caries in humans at present.

6. *Xylitol* This sugar alcohol which cannot be fermented by oral microorganisms is added to some toothpastes in Scandinavia. It sweetens the paste and has an anticaries action by enhancing remineralization and reducing the levels of mutans streptococci.

Mucosal irritation due to dentifrices

A small percentage of individuals are sensitive to some of the ingredients of dentifrices, particularly the aromatic oils. This can be expressed as desquamation or ulceration of the oral mucosa, gingivitis, angular cheilitis, and perioral dermatitis. The practical solution to this problem is for the patient to change to another dentifrice with a different flavour. Ideally, these patients should use a flavourless paste but unfortunately such a toothpaste is not yet commercially available.

8.3 DOES A CLEAN TOOTH DECAY?[3]

A 'clean tooth', i.e. one that is completely free of plaque, will not decay. However, very few individuals can ever completely remove plaque themselves, even under supervision. The toothbrush cannot clean occlusal and interproximal surfaces effectively; yet these are the surfaces most susceptible to caries. Several studies have been carried out on the effect of supervised and unsupervised toothbrushing and flossing. The results showed that although there was a reduction in plaque and gingivitis, caries incidence was not significantly affected. On the other hand, when flossing was performed daily during the school year by professional personnel, there was a significant reduction in the incidence of approximal caries.

Dental personnel were also used in another series of studies involving frequent professional cleaning using the dental engine. The first of these studies was carried out in Sweden by Lindhe *et al.*[4] over a three-year period. In this study the children in the experimental group, aged 7–14 years, received meticulous cleaning with a rotating rubber cup and a fluoride-containing prophylaxis paste once every two weeks in the first two years, the interval extending to four to eight weeks in the third year. These children, together with their parents, were also given oral and written information on the aetiology and prevention of caries and periodontal disease and were given oral hygiene instruction, reinforced at each visit. The children in the control group received conventional dental care which included supervised toothbrushing with a 0.2 per cent sodium fluoride solution once a month. The results were dramatic: during the three-year period the 84 control subjects developed 790 new carious surfaces while the 93 experimental subjects only developed 42 new carious surfaces. The same authors showed equally positive results in an equivalent study on adults. In two other similar studies when the frequency of professional tooth cleaning was reduced to once every three weeks and once a month the results, though significant, were not so pronounced.

However, a study in the UK[5] showed no significant difference in the incidence of caries when the effect of professional prophylaxis alone was tested in a group of 11–12-year-old females over a three-year period. Unlike the Swedish studies, dietary advice was not given and the prophylactic paste did not contain fluoride. Consequently, the effect of the mechanical cleaning alone was tested.

The results of these studies are important in that they suggest that oral hygiene alone, without dietary advice and fluoride, may not be enough to prevent caries. They also show that conventional dental care without dietary advice and patient motivation is ineffective in terms of future caries prevention.

8.3.1 Advice to patients

What advice should we, as clinicians, give our patients regarding oral hygiene and caries? They should be told that by cleaning with a fluoridated toothpaste they will, in fact, be applying fluoride topically and consequently be helping the saliva to remineralize early lesions. When root surfaces are exposed, it is important that they are cleaned meticulously with the appropriate additional cleaning aids since these areas are extremely susceptible to decay. When patients present with carious lesions, disclosing solutions usually show plaque deposits over these areas (Fig. 1.4, p. 6). This can be a powerful motivating tool to demonstrate to the patient the relevance of good plaque control in these areas (see Chapter 9, p. 158).

How frequently should we advise our patients to clean? In a periodontally healthy mouth, meticulous removal of plaque every second day has been shown to be compatible with the maintenance of gingival health. However, the cariogenicity of plaque is more dependent on external factors such as the amount or frequency of sucrose intake, the buffer capacity, and volume of saliva. Consequently, it is not possible to be dogmatic about the ideal regime for the mechanical removal of plaque that would control both dental diseases. Taking all factors into account, it seems that the old rule of brushing twice a day still has merit, together with the recommendation to use additional cleaning aids once a day. In view of current knowledge of plaque pH and caries, it may be advisable to suggest cleaning *before* a meal which may be potentially cariogenic. Brushing at bedtime is also useful since the teeth are particularly vulnerable during sleep, when salivary flow virtually ceases. However, brushing after a pre-bed cariogenic snack cannot be expected to protect the teeth completely.

8.4 CHLORHEXIDINE: A CHEMICAL AGENT FOR PLAQUE CONTROL

Regular daily mechanical removal of plaque by the patient is the established method of plaque control, and sufficiently motivated individuals reach a high level of proficiency. However, for many others, effective removal of plaque by mechanical means is a difficult procedure to master.

Physically and mentally handicapped individuals may have to rely on others for their oral hygiene. It is also painful to use a toothbrush when acute inflammation is present. Consequently, a great deal of research has been directed towards the use of chemical agents which may inhibit or suppress the deposition of plaque.

If it is believed that all plaque bacteria are potentially cariogenic, then the ideal agent must be capable of complete inhibition of plaque and must be used continuously. However, this ideal agent does not exist. Fortunately, elimination of specific microorganisms, for instance mutans streptococci, may 'throw a spanner' in the bacterial ecology and have a useful role to play in caries control. Nevertheless, any chemical agent would have to satisfy the stringent safety requirements for use in the mouth. In particular, it should not induce the emergence of resistant strains of microorganisms nor produce unwelcome side-effects.

Of all the chemical agents for plaque control, chlorhexidine is the most effective and is used as the 'gold standard' to which any new agent is compared. Consequently, it will be covered in detail.

8.4.1 Mechanism of action, dosage, and delivery[6]

Chlorhexidine is an antiseptic belonging to the chemical group of compounds called bisbiguanides which are bactericidal and fungicidal. It has a broad spectrum of activity against Gram-positive and Gram-negative organisms as well as yeasts. The chlorhexidine molecule is cationic, which means it is positively charged, and because of its positive charge, it is attracted to bacterial cell walls which are negatively charged. The bacterial cell wall is then irreversibly damaged with subsequent precipitation of its cytoplasmic components, resulting in cell death. When used in the mouth cationic antiseptics, because of their positive charge, adsorb to dental tissues, to the acidic proteins covering the teeth and oral mucosa and to the proteins in saliva. It is the adsorbed antiseptic on the tooth surface which exerts the bacteriocidal action against organisms attempting to colonize. The success of an antiseptic as a plaque inhibitor depends not only on its antibacterial properties but also on the rate at which it is released from the tooth surface.

Several other cationic antiseptics such as alexidine, cetyl pyridium chloride, benzalkonium chloride, and hexetedine have all been shown to possess antiplaque properties. Of these agents, chlorhexidine has proved to be the most effective since it is released in the mouth up to eight hours after rinsing. It has also been the most thoroughly tested in relation to safety and has been extensively used for over 20 years. Consequently, at the present time, chlorhexidine is the agent which is generally used.

The plaque-inhibiting properties of a chlorhexidine *mouthrinse* were first demonstrated by Löe and Schiött.[7] They showed that, in a group of dental students, by *rinsing for one minute twice a day with 10 ml of a 0.2 per cent solution* of chlorhexidine, plaque deposition and gingivitis could be almost entirely prevented in the absence of oral hygiene. However, in subsequent experiments on unselected subjects, although chlorhexidine was still very effective, its limitations were highlighted. It did not inhibit plaque totally in the average patient. The presence of calculus, overhanging or defective restorations, and periodontal pockets greater than 3 mm reduced its efficacy since these factors would hamper access of the solution to vulnerable sites. Consequently, its effect is greatly enhanced by supra- and subgingival scaling and correction of defective restorations.

Since the original studies using 10 ml of a 0.2 per cent solution as a mouthrinse, various vehicles have been used to deliver the chlorhexidine to the tooth surface. The application of 2–5 ml of a solution at the same concentration but in a *spray* has been tested with good results on a group of handicapped children. This method of delivery has been shown to be very acceptable and is therefore very useful to enable such patients to reach acceptable levels of oral cleanliness. It is also a convenient method of maintaining a clean mouth for debilitated patients or for patients with fixed oral splints. Chlorhexidine is also available in the form of a *gel* at a concentration of 1 per cent. This can be used on a toothbrush or in custom-made vinyl applicator trays (see Fig. 5.2, p. 77).

Chlorhexidine has also been incorporated in a *varnish*. Concentrations of up to 40 per cent have been tested for caries control with positive results, but such high concentrations are unlikely to be licensed for clinical use in the UK. Recently, chlorhexidine at a low concentration of 1 per cent has been incorporated in a varnish together with 1 per cent thymol. Following a prophylaxis, the varnish is applied to the dried and isolated tooth surfaces with a disposable brush in the dental surgery. The material is dispersed with air and the patient may be allowed to rinse. Four hours should elapse before normal oral hygiene. Initial results with this varnish show that mutans streptococci are suppressed for up to three months after treatment and clinical studies to test its cariostatic properties are in progress. If results prove to be positive this regime would take the place of chlorhexidine gel application in trays since it requires no effort on the part of the patient and therefore compliance will not be a problem.

8.4.2 Side-effects

Staining

The most conspicuous side-effect is the development of a yellow/brown stain on the teeth and tongue and on the margins of anterior restorations. Staining around these restorations can be prevented if they are coated with Vaseline before rinsing. The stain is caused by the interaction of chlorhexidine with certain constituents of the diet. It is more severe following mouthrinses and in the absence of toothbrushing and is increased by excessive intake of tea, coffee, red wine, and port. Professional cleaning is required to remove it, but when it accumulates around the margins of defective restorations it is impossible to remove. This limits the long-term use of chlorhexidine.

Taste

Chlorhexidine has a bitter taste and there is a general dulling of taste sensation for a few minutes to several hours after rinsing, depending on the individual. The bitter taste has been masked quite successfully by flavouring agents.

Parotid gland swelling

A few cases of unilateral or bilateral swelling of the parotid glands have been reported. However, they were all reversible when rinsing was discontinued.

Desquamation of oral mucosa

There may be individual variation in the tolerance level of the oral mucosa to chlorhexidine. Consequently a few cases of painful desquamatous lesions have been reported. All cases resolved when rinsing was discontinued or when the mouthwash was diluted 1:1 with water. When the mouthrinse is prescribed for patients whose oral mucosa is compromised due to desquamation or ulceration they should be advised to add water to the original 10 ml dose until it no longer causes stinging. It is also important to instruct the patient to use the total diluted volume to achieve maximum plaque inhibition.

Long-term effects

The effects of two years' regular use of chlorhexidine have been studied.[8] There were no untoward lasting consequences. There is a slight change in the balance of oral flora in favour of the organisms that are less sensitive to it, but this returns to normal after three months. Gingival biopsies taken 18 months after daily use by human subjects showed no histological abnormalities.

8.5 THE USE OF CHLORHEXIDINE IN THE CONTROL OF CARIES[9]

Much of the original work on chlorhexidine was directed towards the control of plaque microorganisms implicated in gingivitis and periodontal disease. However, because of its broad spectrum of activity, chlorhexidine is equally effective against mutans streptococci, the prime pathogen in the initiation of caries. In an experimental caries model using dental students, it was demonstrated that rinsing nine times daily with 50 per cent sucrose did not result in caries when the students also rinsed twice a day with 10 ml of a 0.2 per cent solution of chlorhexidine. A more recent study showed that it was possible to control caries in a group of children with a high caries incidence and high salivary mutans streptococci levels by the use of a chlorhexidine gel. In this study a 1 per cent chlorhexidine gel in custom-made applicators was used for five minutes daily for 14 days every four months if the salivary mutans streptococci counts exceeded 2.5×10^5 per ml. This regime was also shown to be effective in reducing high levels of mutans streptococci in mothers and in interfering in the transmission of these organisms to their infants. Using a similar regime supplemented with a daily fluoride mouth rinse, caries was successfully controlled in patients who had received radiotherapy in the head and neck region and were therefore highly susceptible to caries.[10]

Chlorhexidine and fluoride have also been combined in a single mouth-wash or solution for topical application and tested with some success both in children and adults. These studies show that fluoride and chlorhexidine are compatible. Unfortunately, at the moment chlorhexidine/fluoride solutions or gels are not available commercially.

8.5.1 Indications

Since there is sufficient evidence to show that chlorhexidine is a very effective plaque inhibitor, should its daily use be advocated for everyone in order to control caries? The long term unsupervised daily use of any such anti-microbial is contraindicated because of the possible development of resistant strains of organisms. In addition the side-effects of chlorhexidine, particularly staining, would preclude its use routinely. Furthermore, plaque is not always cariogenic. Indeed, even though mutans streptococcus is a prime pathogen in dental caries, its presence in the mouth is not always indicative of caries susceptibility.

The use of chlorhexidine as an anticaries agent should be considered only for those individuals who have been assessed to be 'at high risk' to active caries (see Chapter 4). This assessment should be made on the basis of history, clinical and radiographic examination, dietary history, salivary secretion rate, and buffer capacity. In most cases dietary control, good oral hygiene, and topically applied fluoride (varnish or rinse) are adequate to control caries. However, if these measures have failed, or if caries is rampant, chlorhexidine should be used as outlined below.

Patients with greatly reduced salivary flow, who are consequently very much 'at risk' to caries, benefit from the prophylactic use of chlorhexidine in conjunction with fluoride (see Section 5.4). In the future, if more evidence becomes available, chlorhexidine may also be used prophylactically to prevent the transmission of cariogenic microorganisms from parents to children and from primary teeth to the permanent dentition.

8.5.2 Method of application

Before application, all open carious lesions should be restored or dressed. A prophylaxis will reduce subsequent staining. Flexible vinyl applicator trays (see Fig. 5.2, p. 77) are made for each patient for self-application of a 1 per cent gel for five minutes daily for 14 days. About five to ten drops of the gel are spread evenly in each tray. During application, chewing movements by the patient will ensure that the gel reaches interproximal areas. This form of application is more comfortable and more effective than rinsing with a solution or brushing with a gel since it is not diluted by saliva and is confined to the teeth. Consequently, the tongue and mucous membranes have little contact with it, minimizing mucosal irritation and alteration of taste sensation. After gel application the mouth should be rinsed with water.

It is important to note that chlorhexidine is inactivated by sodium lauryl sulphate, the detergent present in most toothpastes. Patients should therefore be instructed to rinse toothpaste out thoroughly before any chlorhexidine application.

The effects of chlorhexidine used in this way for the control of caries should be monitored by microbiological examination. If it has been successful in reducing the salivary mutans streptococci counts to below 2.5×10^5 per ml, the patient should continue to use a daily fluoride mouthrinse to help remineralize any chalky enamel lesions. If the count remains high, the patient has probably not used the gel as directed. In such cases it may be possible to reduce the mutans streptococci counts by applying the gel in the surgery for three five-minute applications on two consecutive days, allowing the patient to rinse with water between applications.

In some cases recolonization may occur due to remnants of mutans streptococcus in cracks in the enamel surface or in patients with dry mouth as a result of radiotherapy (see Section 5.4.3). Consequently, retreatment may be necessary every three to four months. In every case dietary advice and oral hygiene instruction must precede treatment with chlorhexidine.

8.6 OTHER CHEMICAL AGENTS FOR PLAQUE CONTROL[11]

Four main groups of chemical agents other than chlorhexidine have been investigated: enzymes, surface active agents, antibiotics, and antibacterial agents.

8.6.1 Enzymes

Hydrolytic, proteolytic, and glycolytic enzymes have been tested in attempts to break down the plaque matrix and so cause disruption and dispersal of the plaque. So far these attempts have proved ineffective or impractical due to the complex nature of the intermicrobial matrix of dental plaque and the specificity and short duration of action of some of these enzymes. Problems concerning the potential toxicity of some of the preparations tested were also encountered.

Another approach is to use enzymes to enhance the antibacterial properties of saliva. However, the addition of the enzymes amyloglucosidase and glucose oxidase to mouthwashes and toothpastes has produced conflicting results (see Section 8.2.5).

8.6.2 Surface-active agents

Theoretically it is an attractive proposition to alter the tooth surface so that it becomes difficult for plaque to adhere. Studies *in vitro* show that fluoride may be capable of retarding the deposition of pellicle and plaque although there is little evidence *in vivo* to support this.

Attempts have been made to form moisture-repellent coatings on the smooth surfaces of teeth. Silicones and sulfonated polystyrene have been tested with no success. Preliminary studies using the amine-substituted alcohols (octapinol and delmopinol) have been encouraging. With the great strides being made in the field of dental materials we may, indeed, be able to look forward to a successful plaque-repellent coating.

8.6.3 Antibiotics

Penicillin, tetracycline, spiramycin, and erythromycin have all been shown to inhibit plaque formation. A study involving children with rheumatic fever, who were taking large systemic doses of penicillin to prevent streptococcal infection, showed a 55 per cent reduction in caries after two years. However, such antibiotics are important for the treatment of more serious infections so that the potential dangers associated with sensitization and the development of resistant strains of organisms as well as superinfection by fungal organisms prohibit their use for routine plaque control.

8.6.4 Antibacterial agents

Fluoride

The effect of fluoride on plaque bacteria and bacterial metabolism has been discussed (see Section 7.3). Loesche et al.[12] showed that the use of ten topical applications of APF (1.23 per cent acidulated phosphate fluoride) over a 10-day period resulted in a 70 per cent reduction in the level of mutans streptococci present in dental plaque. Whilst this demonstrates the antibacterial action of fluoride, the daily home use of fluoride at such a high concentration cannot be generally recommended because of safety considerations (see Section 7.8). Although lower concentrations of fluoride can affect bacterial metabolism, the bactericidal effect of the concentrations used in dentifrices and mouthwashes remains to be confirmed.

Triclosan

Triclosan has a broad spectrum of antimicrobial activity against yeasts and Gram-positive and Gram-negative bacteria. It has been added to mouthwashes and toothpastes (see Section 8.2.5) together with zinc citrate and a co-polymer. Although it has been shown to reduce plaque deposition and gingivitis to some extent, its value as a cariostatic agent is not yet proven adequately.

Metal ions

Zinc, tin, and copper have shown some antiplaque activity. Zinc citrate enhances the action of triclosan and zinc, tin, and copper have also shown cariostatic effects in rats. Adverse reactions related to clinical use are an unpleasant metal taste with a feeling of dryness and some staining.

REFERENCES

1. Marsh, P. and Martin, H. (1992). *Oral microbiology*, (3rd edn), Ch. 6: Dental caries. Chapman & Hall, London.

2. Murray, J. J., Rugg-Gunn, A., and Jenkins, G.N. (1991). *Fluorides in caries prevention*, (3rd edn), Ch 9: Fluoride toothpastes and dental caries. Butterworth-Heinemann, Oxford.

3. Thylstrup, A. and Fejerskov, O. (1994). *Textbook of clinical cariology*, (2nd edn), Ch. 10: Oral hygiene and dental caries. Munksgaard, Copenhagen.

4. Lindhe, J., Axelsson, P., and Tollskog, G. (1975). Effect of proper oral hygiene on gingivitis and dental caries in Swedish schoolchildren. *Community Dent. Oral Epidemiol*, **3**, 150–5.

5. Ashley, F.P. and Sainsbury, R.H. (1981). The effect of a school-based plaque control programme on caries and gingivitis. *Br. Dent. J.*, **150**, 4l–5.

6. Löe, H. (1973). Symposium on chlorhexidine in the prophylaxis of dental diseases. *J. Periodont. Res*, suppl. no. 12, **8**, 5–99.

7. Löe, H. and Schiött, C.R. (1970). The effect of mouthrinses and topical application of chlorhexidine on the development of dental plaque and gingivitis in man. *J. Periodont. Res*, **5**, 79–83.

8. Löe, H. (ed) (1976). Two years oral use of chlorhexidine in man. *J. Periodont. Res*, **11**, 135–75.

9. Kidd, E.A.M. (1991). The role of chlorhexidine in the management of dental caries. *Int. Dent. J.*, **41**, 279–86.

10. Joyston-Bechal, S., Hayes, K., Davenport, E., and Hardie, J.M. (1992). Caries, mutans streptococci and lactobacilli in irradiated patients during a 12 month programme using chlorhexidine and fluoride. *Caries Res.*, **26**, 384–90.

11. Embery, G. and Rolla, G. (1992). *Clinical and biological aspect of dentifrices*, Ch. 18: Mechanism of action of clinically proven anti-plaque agents. Oxford University Press.

12. Loesche, W.J., Syed, R.J., Murray, R.J., and Mellberg, J. (1975). The effect of topical acidulated fluoride on percentage of *Streptococcus mutans* and *Streptococcus sanguis* in plaque. *Caries Res.*, **9**, 139–55.

9

Patient motivation*

9.1 THE ESSENTIAL ROLE OF THE PATIENT

The last three chapters have discussed the management of dental caries by control of diet, the use of fluoride supplements at home, and the removal of plaque by the patient. The success of all these strategies depends on the patient, but it is a well known fact that patients frequently

*This chapter is written by Teresa Barker.

choose not to comply with health advice given to them. Many know they should lose weight, take more exercise, finish their course of antibiotics, practise 'safe' sex, give up smoking, but choose not to. Although exact levels of compliance are difficult to measure, it has been estimated that one-third to one-half of all patients fail to follow fully the advice given to them.[1]

A lot of time and effort is spent on giving advice to patients, and this is costly. If the advice is seemingly ignored by the patient it can lead to frustration and increasing dissatisfaction for members of the dental team, quite apart from the fact that the patient's disease level remains unaltered.

Throughout the text it has been stated that the carious process can be modified by altering diet, use of fluoride, and improved plaque control. It is the patient who has the essential role here. It is therefore important to understand fully the subject of patient motivation and behaviour change before offering any preventive advice. The preventive treatment required should be planned by the dentist who may delegate some tasks to a therapist, a hygienist, or a dental health educator. In this chapter the operator is often referred to as 'the dentist' but the chapter is equally applicable to the other members of the dental team.

9.2 DEFINITION OF MOTIVATION

To motivate is to stimulate the interest of a person, causing them to act. There has been much misunderstanding surrounding patient motivation and it has often erroneously been thought of as either simply telling a patient what to do and telling them again if they have not complied the first time or as a simple technique of forcing them to change their behaviour. The old saying, 'You can lead a horse to water but you cannot make it drink' is apt, and a useful reminder that motivation is about creating the desire within another to want to follow advice for their own benefit. It has been suggested that patients may be divided into three broad groups: those who are naturally well motivated, others who possess 'latent' motivation who just require the right stimulus at the right time, and a third group who often appear impossible to motivate.[2]

The following case may illustrate this. A 25-year-old male patient could not be persuaded to brush his teeth more than once a month. Much time and effort was spent in attempting to get him to change his behaviour but he continued to attend for his hygienist appointments with a month's growth of plaque. On one of the final appointments he said he had recently married. Seizing the opportunity, the hygienist, in a final attempt to motivate this patient to change his behaviour, asked 'What do you think it is like for your wife when you only clean your teeth once a month?'. At the next appointment there was not a scrap of plaque to be seen. He was brushing twice a day and needed no further persuasion!

9.3 FACTORS AFFECTING PATIENT MOTIVATION

9.3.1 Whose problem?

'It isn't that they can't see the solution, it's that they can't see the problem'
The Scandal of Father Brown
G.K. Chesterton

This is not a reference to dental patients but it summarizes the problem well. Many people are ignorant about dental disease and do not recognize it as a problem. This is partly an indictment on our role as educators. Many patients think that it is the dentist's responsibility to care for their mouths. However, in a year a dentist may only see a patient for two hours out of the total 8760. Since plaque re-forms every 24 hours, its removal has to be the responsibility of the patient. It is vital that patients recognize and acknowledge this and therefore the dental team must take time to talk and listen to them.

Many people have grown up with the idea that it is inevitable and normal to need fillings and even lose teeth. A middle-aged patient, on being told he had five new holes in his teeth remarked 'Well that's not bad is it— after all I am 45 so I've done pretty well to have kept my teeth as long as this, haven't I?'. Such a patient is accepting and unconcerned about on-going disease in his mouth. Attempts at motivation stand a greater chance of success if the dentist first shares his or her concern and then finds out what level of concern, if any, the patient has. This is an important starting place and will guide the dentist as to how to proceed. It will prevent premature and apparently irrelevant advice being given.

9.3.2 Patients' beliefs

It must not be taken for granted that a patient holds the same beliefs as the dentist. This is illustrated by the following case. A patient with seven new carious cavities and several early white spot lesions was instructed on the first appointment to buy a fluoride mouthwash for daily use. On the second appointment he was asked how he was getting on with it, and it turned out he wasn't using it. Therefore, the instructions given on the first appointment were repeated, at length. On the third appointment he was again asked how he was getting on with the fluoride mouthwash and he again replied that he hadn't started using it. Instructions were about to be repeated for the third time when the hygienist stopped and asked the patient if he believed fluoride helped to prevent holes. 'No', replied the patient.

It is important to take time to find out what patients believe, because this will affect the advice given and subsequently compliance. In this case time and effort should have been spent attempting to modify the patient's beliefs.

9.3.3 Personally relevant advice

If patients are to change their behaviour they must see the advice offered as being relevant to them. It is easy to give every patient the same advice, such as how to brush and floss, the importance of dietary control of sugar, and use of a fluoride mouthrinse. However, it is important that the advice is tailored to the individual needs of the patient. For example there is no point in persuading a 50-year-old patient to complete a diet analysis sheet if examination reveals that caries is not a current problem.

9.3.4 Enthusiasm

A salesperson who strongly believes in the product engenders enthusiasm and interest in the potential purchaser. 'Selling' the concept of dental health to a patient has a greater chance of success if the dentist promotes 'the product' with enthusiasm. Words such as 'This small headed brush will really help you to get to those back teeth and you'll notice they no longer feel furred up but shiny and clean' encourage a patient to feel spending extra time on plaque removal is worthwhile.

9.3.5 High trust—low fear

Trust between dentist and patient often develops over time. It is in a high-trust environment that patients are more likely to follow advice so it is important to continue to develop a good relationship so that trust increases with each visit. The response that the dentist hopes for may take several years of patience and understanding.

When patients are slow to follow advice, it may be tempting to resort to threatening them with the consequences. Studies[3] have shown that while the use of fear and threat may produce behaviour change, this is limited to the short term. Fear and threat should therefore be used cautiously. 'I am concerned about the number of new cavities you have in your teeth' may be a much better approach than 'If you don't follow my advice you are going to lose all your teeth by the time you're 60'!

9.3.6 Care

If the dentist can convey to the patient that they care about them and have a genuine interest in their dental health, compliance is more likely. So to say to a patient who is struggling with dental floss 'It looks as though you find that extremely awkward to use' lets the patient know you understand their difficulties. The dentist can then offer alternatives, such as bottle brushes, which the patient may find easier to use.

9.3.7 Praise

Praise is a strong motivator and patients respond positively to this, whereas rebuke demotivates them. One patient was heard to remark that he gave up trying to brush better because no matter how hard he tried, his efforts were constantly criticized. Even if there is only a slight improvement or a small change in behaviour it is important to acknowledge this in a positive way. This can be done by saying 'I can see you have put a lot of effort into your brushing and the gums look very much better around your front teeth'. After this, further advice can be offered in the areas where there is still room for improvement.

9.3.8 Negotiation

Szasz and Hollender[4] state that there are three types of relationship that may exist between patients and health professionals:

1. **The active–passive** relationship where the dentist assumes total responsibility for the patient who remains passive in the encounter. A patient having a general anaesthetic would be an example of this.
2. **The guidance–cooperation** relationship where the dentist is seen as the 'expert' who gives advice with which the patient is expected to comply.
3. **The mutual participation** relationship where the dentist and the patient share equally. The patient's thoughts, ideas, and beliefs are considered as important as the dentist's advice and technical expertise. This relationship is the most appropriate to motivate patients to adopt

preventive health behaviours. Thus there is a greater chance of a patient following health advice if negotiation has taken place.

For example if the dentist feels the patient should cut out sugar in drinks and use an artificial sweetener instead, it would be best to negotiate with the patient rather than dictate to them. A question such as 'How would you feel about trying to give up sugar in tea and coffee?' or 'What would you feel about trying an artificial sweetener?' would be ways of negotiating with a patient. This provides them with the opportunity to share their beliefs or ideas which are important because these attitudes affect compliance.

Patients will often comment that they do not like the taste of artificial sweeteners and would therefore find it hard to change their habits. In this situation, it is helpful to make a number of cups of tea for the patient sweetened with various artificial sweeteners and one cup sweetened with sugar. Each cup should be designated by a letter and the patient asked to rank the acceptability of the drink with marks out of ten. Surprisingly, some patients cannot recognize sugar and will give one of the artificial sweeteners an equal ranking. This demonstration can aid the negotiation and be a powerful motivating tool, encouraging the patient to buy the appropriate sugar substitute.

9.3.9 Realistic goals

With an enthusiastic approach to motivation it is easy to set a patient unrealistic goals without appreciating their point of view. For example, a patient who is told to brush for half an hour a day will not comply with this advice because it is totally unrealistic. If the patient is included in the negotiation (see Section 9.3.8) it is likely that a realistic goal will be set. For instance if a dentist would like a patient to floss, the importance of flossing should be discussed and the technique demonstrated in one part of the mouth— perhaps on an approximal surface where an enamel lesion is present on radiograph. The patient can be asked how often it would be realistic to floss this contact. If the patient suggests flossing the area twice a week, this should be accepted as a realistic goal. In learning any new skill it is important to build in small steps. At subsequent visits, dentist and patient may together decide to move the goal posts, perhaps by agreeing to floss the same area daily or by including other susceptible contact points.

9.3.10 Regular positive reinforcement and follow-up

Maintaining changes in behaviour in the long term is difficult. Broken New Year resolutions are an obvious example. It is therefore important that a patient's progress is followed up regularly, and positive reinforcement offered where they have maintained changes in their behaviour. For example, where agreement to try an artificial sweetener in place of sugar was reached on the first appointment, an opening gambit on the second appointment could be 'How have you got on with the artificial sweetener?'. At a three month review appointment the patient should be asked whether the artificial sweetener is still being used. This encourages the patient to maintain the change.

For the dentist to be able to check how the patient is progressing on subsequent appointments it is important that the notes are fully written up after each visit so that they can be referred to before the next appointment. The notes may say for example:

Patient has agreed to:
1.   Buy fluoride mouthrinse and use daily.
2.   Floss contact /56 twice a week.
3.   Complete diet sheet and return it next visit.

These agreed goals should also be written down at the end of the appointment for the patient to take away because it is easy to forget or misinterpret what was agreed. The notes also provide the dentist with a good starting point on the next visit. 'Did you manage to buy the fluoride mouthrinse after your last visit?' and also provide the opportunity to offer positive reinforcement to encourage the patient.

A record can also be kept of any aspect of the patient's social history that may be useful. A patient was amazed and pleased when his dentist asked at a six month follow-up appointment 'Have you started outdoor bowls yet this year?'. The patient commented what an excellent memory the dentist had. In fact it was because the dentist **hadn't** got a good memory that he had made a note of the patient's hobby. Comments such as these can help to build relationships with patients and enhance motivation.

9.3.11 Scoring

A scoring system that enables both dentist and patient to monitor behaviour change may be helpful. For instance a simple system of scoring plaque may be used. If the patient is told that an acceptable plaque score is around 10 per cent and after disclosing he or she learns the score is a lot higher than this, the effect can be to encourage further effort. At the next appointment the patient's opening remarks are often 'What's my score today? I've worked hard at trying to get it down since I last saw you.'

9.4 COMMUNICATION

An ability to communicate is central to achieving behaviour change. A well known quotation highlights some of the problems encountered in communication. 'I know you **believe** you understand what you **think** I said, but I am not sure you realise that what you **heard** is not what I meant.'[5]

There is a tendency to think that because we learn to speak from an early age (and on average we each use up to 5000 words per day), communication is not a skill that can be learnt or improved upon once we become adults. Just as the ability to do operative dentistry is learnt, practised, and perfected, so it is with communication skills.

The work of Mehrabian[6] suggests that communication is made up of three parts:

- 7 per cent *actual words* conveying information
- 38 per cent *tone* conveying emotions and attitudes
- 55 per cent *non-verbal communication* also conveying emotions and attitudes.

Understanding the relative importance of these components may explain why communication sometimes breaks down and why patients often appear unmotivated and non-compliant. These components will now be considered in more detail.

9.4.1 Actual words

The following factors can affect the success of communication in the verbal channel:.

1. *Dental jargon.* Patients frequently misunderstand common dental words. 'Plaque', 'caries', and 'bacteria' may well be words the patient has heard frequently but may not know their real meaning. Information should be given simply and it is not unreasonable to check a patient's understanding by asking a question such as 'Can you tell me what you understand by the term plaque?'. Some patients think plaque is calculus and therefore the dentist's responsibility to remove and not theirs.

Words chosen in giving explanations will vary according to the knowledge and expectations of the listener. The listener should be neither belittled nor befuddled by the message. Explaining the cause of caries to a chemistry graduate will differ from the explanation offered to a child.

2. *Listening.* Research suggests that we only listen at 25 per cent of our full potential.[7] The patient may be anxious about dental treatment or have other pressing things on the mind such as collecting the children from

school or an important business meeting. Thus information given is not always received, remembered, or acted upon.

To overcome this, advice and instructions should be given early in an appointment with the most important point being stressed, and then repeated as the patient leaves the surgery. As stated in Section 9.3.10, if the instructions are also written down the patient has less chance of forgetting or distorting what was agreed. The dentist's message to a caries-prone patient at the beginning of the appointment may be 'To prevent further holes in your teeth it is going to be very important for you to reduce the number of sugar "attacks" you have each day.' This can be restated as the patient leaves the surgery as 'So we've agreed the most important thing you are going to do is to try an artificial sweetener in your tea and coffee to cut down the sugar "attacks".'

It is important that the dentist listens to what the patient has to say. We are also guilty of listening with only a half or even a quarter of an ear to our patients. A study showed that doctors interrupted their patients after a mean time of 18 seconds.[8] A study of dentists would no doubt reveal a similar pattern. A recent leader in the British Medical Journal posed the question 'What do patients want?' and cited evidence that patients want someone who will listen to them.[9]

3. *Forgetting.* Patients forget advice more than other types of information and it is suggested that 50 per cent of information given is forgotten within five minutes of a patient leaving the surgery.[10] It is important not to overload the patient with information as three or four key points are the most they are likely to remember at one appointment.

4. *Distortion.* There is a tendency to distort what we have heard and to put our own interpretation on it. Patients taught the Bass technique of brushing may return brushing vigorously using the 'up and down' technique believing they are following the dentist's advice. Dietary advice also gets distorted. A 12-year-old girl with a high caries rate was advised to stop drinking squash containing sugar and to buy sugar-free squash instead. Her father, who brought her for her dental appointment agreed that they would do this. Written instructions were given to the parents. A subsequent phone conversation with the girl's mother some weeks later elicited that they had purchased a 'reduced sugar' squash which unfortunately was also cariogenic.

9.4.2 Tone

Tone conveys attitudes and emotions such as enthusiasm or boredom. Patients will soon detect these emotions from the dentist's tone of voice and while enthusiasm is infectious, boredom is demotivating. Dentists can also detect a patient's emotions from the tone of their voice. When this tone indicates a message has not been well received it is worth trying to discuss the matter further. A comment from the dentist such as 'I don't think I've convinced you', may open the door to exploring the perceived difficulty with the patient.

9.4.3 Non-verbal communication or body language

Facial expression

One of the main functions of facial expression is to communicate emotions and attitudes and it may be that a dentist will know a patient has no intention of following advice given just by observing the patient's facial expression. The patient will also pick up the facial expression of the dentist which may inadvertently register judgement, disapproval, disbelief, or even dislike. This can affect communication and ultimately motivation. Conversely facial expression can be used to enhance motivation. Something as simple as a smile helps to put patients at their ease and enhance trust. In a particularly unpleasant experiment[11] the facial muscles of some infant monkeys and their mothers were cut and it was found that the pairs failed to develop any relationship with each other.

Eye contact

Eye contact is important because it enables both the dentist and the patient to collect information which can be used to guide the way the consultation is going. Students report feeling very frustrated when patients gaze out of the window whilst they are talking to them and will not give them eye contact. They say 'I've no idea if they are listening to me or not—I don't know whether to go on or to stop.' When advice is being offered, ensure that the patient is seated at the same level as the dentist and not lying supine. If the patient continues to avoid eye contact, stop talking and wait to see what effect this has. If this fails, acknowledge that the patient does not appear to be listening and say 'You seem uninterested in what I am saying. Is there a reason for this?' This should bring eye contact back and provide the opportunity for the patient to explain what they are finding difficult.

To know how it feels to be a patient, try lying in the dental chair, and attempt to floss or brush watching yourself in a mirror held by a colleague who is also giving you advice. All eye contact is lost and there is a sense of being 'talked down to' and a strong feeling of disempowerment.

Gestures and bodily movements

When emotions are aroused, pointless bodily movements are often made. For example, an anxious patient may scratch their neck or adjust their jacket or skirt. A patient unwilling to state that he or she has not used the fluoride mouthwash recommended at the last visit may, for example, brush imaginary fluff from their sleeve when asked about mouthwash use.

Bodily posture

Posture can communicate as clearly as words. If the dentist is running late, and the patient in the waiting is room standing with their hands on their hips and chin thrust forward, this communicates a warning to 'proceed with caution!'. When running late it is wise to inform the patient of the delay and apologize for it. Starting with an immediate apology will usually defuse a potentially explosive situation.

Bodily contact

Argyle[12] points out that bodily contact in our culture is controlled by strict rules and is used mainly by families and courting couples. Professionals such as doctors and dentists use it, but not as a social act. In dentistry the adult patient usually accepts without question that their visit will involve touch but it should be remembered that bodily contact can also help or hinder communication. A firm handshake in greeting may increase a patient's confidence in their dentist but not all students feel comfortable doing this or indeed think that it is always necessary or appropriate. A hand on the shoulder of an anxious patient as the dental chair is taken back may convey care for the patient and be reassuring to those who are anxious but a confident patient may feel patronized or annoyed by it. Each case needs to be assessed individually.

Spatial behaviour

In most walks of life the importance of personal space is recognized and respected, apart from situations where overcrowding is accepted as normal, such as lifts and crowded public transport. Four spatial zones have been suggested[13] and these are:

- intimate zone,   15–50 cm
- personal zone,   50 cm–1.2 m
- social zone,   1.2–3.6 m
- public zone,   3.6 m.

The personal space referred to as the 'intimate zone' is usually reserved for close friends but when a dentist examines or operates it is automatically invaded. This is accepted by patients but it is worth remembering that for some patients there may be some embarrassment and anxiety that affects them receiving the dentist's communication in this 'intimate zone'. Kent[14] states that just because it is culturally acceptable it should not be taken to be without meaning for the patient. When giving advice to a patient it is a good idea to return the dental chair to the upright position, ensure that eye contact is on the same level and move away from the patient to a position where communication is comfortable for both parties.

Clothes and appearance

Clothes and appearance communicate information. A white coat for example may communicate one thing to a patient whereas a blue or green coat may communicate something different. One study showed that children's heart rates increased by 10 beats per minute when a dentist put on a white coat.[15] Badges too communicate information. The paediatric dentist who wears a teddy bear badge is communicating a message to a child patient and to the parent.

The style and decor of the surgery and waiting room also communicate a message to patients. Dental students who were asked to rate the skill and competence of several hypothetical dentists by looking at photographs of old fashioned, modern, and ultra-modern surgeries, inferred that a dentist with an ultra-modern surgery would be more trustworthy, more skilful and more competent.[16] Something as simple as plants, lighting, types and states of magazines all communicate, albeit at a subconscious level. One patient, when asked what she thought of the dentist's waiting room, pointed to the posters on the walls displaying pictures of bad gums and teeth and said 'Tell the dentist to take those home and put them on his sitting room wall and bring us in the pictures he's got hanging there instead.'

9.5 FACTORS WHICH ENHANCE LEARNING

9.5.1 Involve the patient

'Tell me and I forget
Show me and I remember
Involve me and I learn'

Confucius, circa 500BC

When the dentist hopes to motivate a patient to comply with health advice it is not enough just to tell them or show them, there is also a need to involve them. This can be done in the surgery in a number of ways such as:

1. ask the patient to brush or floss during oral hygiene instruction;
2. show them an extracted decayed tooth or their own radiograph;
3. encourage them to feel a piece of calculus you have removed from their teeth;
4. offer them a sugar free mint to taste;
5. ask them to take away and complete a diet analysis sheet.

9.5.2 Make use of other senses

There is a tendency to rely only on verbal communication forgetting that sight, sound, touch, taste, and smell can all be used in motivation. More material can be retained if more than one sense is used to receive information. Thus to involve a patient's senses of sight, hearing, and touch in learning anything new, is likely to bring about a greater retention of material than if only one of these senses is used.

It is not difficult to involve senses other than hearing. For instance when teaching a patient to use a toothbrush the dentist may place a hand over the patient's hand to guide their movement. The patient will *feel* the brush touching the gingivae and *hear* how little noise is made by the brush when the Bass technique is correctly carried out. Ineffective scrubbing with a brush is noisy but effective insertion of the filaments interdentally and vibratory movement is quiet. The patient may also *see* blood on the filaments. It is important to explain that this is a consequence of inflammation and does not imply the patient has been rough. Finally, the patient can be encouraged to run their tongue over the teeth to *feel* the shiny, smooth surface of plaque-free teeth. Similarly the senses can be used when teaching a patient to floss. The patient may be able to *see* plaque on the floss, *smell* the putrid odour of plaque removed from a stagnation area, and *feel* calculus obstructing free movement of the floss.

9.5.3 Amount of information given

Patients are unlikely to remember more than three or four key points at any one appointment. It is sensible to give less information rather than more and check that it has been understood. Many patients, either wishing to please or trying to avoid looking foolish, will nod readily when listening to

advice being given but often have not really understood. Sometimes understanding can be checked. For instance if a fluoride mouthwash has been
recommended, at the end of the appointment the patient could be asked to
use it. This is not to 'catch the patient out' but to help the dentist see if the
message given earlier has been understood and give help if necessary.

9.5.4 Short, simple, and specific advice

Most of us find it difficult to remember complex and lengthy explanations of
subjects which are not our particular speciality. Advice to patients has a
greater chance of being retained and acted upon if it is kept short, simple,
and specific. So to say to a patient with early white spot lesions 'You have
several white spot lesions and early areas of demineralization which may
respond to a regime of fluoride therapy', would not be helpful. To say,
however, 'There are lots of new holes starting in your teeth. I would like
you to use a fluoride mouthrinse daily to try and prevent them from getting
any worse' gets the message home simply and clearly.

9.5.5 Timing

Timing of preventive advice is important. For example it will not be well
received by a patient in pain. However, once toothache has been relieved
preventive treatment may be accepted as relevant to prevent recurrence of
the problem.

Preventive advice should not be relegated to the end of an appointment
because the patient may be tired and anxious to leave. Operative and preventive treatment may be combined in one appointment but the preventive
element requires maximum patient participation and should be carried out
first. Some preventive items take longer than others. The time for a local
anaesthetic to work may be sufficient to show a patient how to use a
mouthwash. Dietary analysis and advice is more time consuming and may
require a separate appointment.

It is surprising how often students will scale a quadrant and *then* give
oral hygiene instruction. This is illogical since the plaque that the patient
should see will have been removed. Oral hygiene instruction should precede
scaling. However, even this rule is made to be broken sometimes. It may be
helpful for a patient with very heavy plaque and calculus deposits to have
one quadrant professionally cleaned before oral hygiene instruction so that
they can see and feel the difference this has made.

Social history is often relevant to the timing of preventive treatment. For
instance, flossing is time consuming. When does the patient have the time

to do this? It is sensible to discuss this and let the patient suggest the appropriate time.

9.6 FAILURE

It would be nice to think that if all the advice in this chapter was followed, failures in patient motivation would never occur. This is not the case. It was stated in Section 9.1 that one-third to one-half of all patients fail to follow fully the advice given to them. This may be for all manner of reasons, many of which have been discussed in this chapter. If you feel you have failed to motivate a patient it is worth asking yourself, in the light of the contents of this chapter, if there is anything you could or should have done differently.

Some psychological theories may throw additional light on issues of non-compliance. The *health belief model*[17] states that for an individual to take action they have to believe they are susceptible to the disease, that the disease is serious, and the benefits of following the prescribed advice out-weigh the costs. Many patients may not believe caries is serious or that they are susceptible to it. For some patients the cost of spending extra time in the bathroom flossing and rinsing with a fluoride mouthwash outweigh any perceived benefit and this may explain why they have not followed the advice given.

The health locus of control theory[17] states that individuals hold beliefs about whether they have any control over what happens to them. They may have a fatalistic approach 'Teeth just rot; there's nothing I can do about it.' This demonstrates an external locus of control where the patient believes fate or chance are in control. They may say 'It's the dentist's responsibility to care for my mouth, not mine' demonstrating an external locus of control where the patient believes 'powerful others' are in control of what happens. Conversely, they may have an internal locus of control and say 'I believe I can prevent further holes in my teeth'. The latter patient will not be hard to motivate but the two former examples will need all the educator's enthusiasm, patience, and skill.

The theory of reasoned action[18] states that an individual will only perform a certain behaviour if they perceive it is worthwhile and if others who are significant to them also believe the same thing. Thus a teenage patient who the dentist tries to persuade to attend for regular check ups may not comply because they are influenced by their peer group who do not believe regular dental attendance is worthwhile. Similarly a patient whose family members have false teeth with which they are quite happy may not listen to the attempts of the educator to persuade them to give up sugar in drinks in order to prevent them from finishing up with false teeth. If the reader is interested in these psychological models they are referred to a text which deals with them in more detail.[18]

The importance of the dental team should not be underestimated in patient motivation. What the dentist may not be able to achieve, the hygienist, nurse, or dental health educator may, or vice versa. Sometimes it can be something as simple as a different personality taking over which changes the outcome.

Motivation of patients can be a slow process. It does not usually happen after one visit. It is often a continuous process of building up trust and rapport with a patient over many visits, continuing to be encouraging and finding small improvements that the educator can be positive about. It is also an ethical necessity to be honest with patients and there will be times when we will have to confront the patient and tell them their preventive efforts are insufficient to prevent dental disease.

As dental health educators we need to remember we can lead a horse to water but we can't make it drink. Ours is the business of creating the environment that makes the 'horse' thirsty.

REFERENCES

1. Kirscht, J.P. and Rosenstock, I.M. (1979). Patients' problems in following recommendations of health experts. In Health psychology, (ed. G.C. Stone, F. Cohen, and N. Adler,) Jossey-Bass, San Francisco.
2. Walsh, T.F.A. (1979). Scientific basis for motivation in dentistry. *Dent. Health*, **18**, 21–7.
3. Janis, I. L. and Feshbach, S. (1953). Effects of fear-arousing communications. *J. Abnorm. Psychol.*, **48**, 78.
4. Szasz T.S. and Hollender M.H. (1956). A contribution to the philosophy of medicine: the basic models of the doctor–patient relationship. *Arch. Intern. Med.*, **97**, 585–92.
5. Geboy, M.J. (1985). Poem attributed to the Religious Public Relations Council. In *Communication and behaviour management in dentistry*. Williams and Wilkins.
6. Mehrabian, A. (1971). *Silent messages*. Wadsworth, Belmont, California.
7. Carkhuff, R.R. (1969). *Helping and human relations: A primer for lay and professional helpers*. Holt, Rinehart, and Winston, New York.
8. Beckman, H.B. and Frankel, R.M. (1984). The effect of physician behaviour on the collection of data. *Ann. Intern. Med*, **101**, 692–6.
9. Armstrong, D. (1991). What do patients want? *Br. Med. J.*, **303**, 203–4.
10. Ley, P., Bradshaw, P.W., Eaves, D., and Walker, C.M. (1973). A method for increasing patients' recall of information presented doctors. *Psychol. Med.*, **3**, 217–20.
11. Izard, C.E. (1975). Patterns of emotions and emotion communication in 'hostility' and aggression. In *Nonverbal communication of aggression*, (ed. P. Pliner, L. Kramer and T. Alloway). Plenum, New York.

12. Argyle, M. (1983). *The psychology of interpersonal behaviour*. Penguin, Harmondsworth.
13. Hall, E.T. (1967). *The hidden dimension*. Bodley Head, London .
14. Kent, G.G. and Blinkhorn, A.S. (1991). *The psychology of dental care*, (2nd edn). Wright, Oxford.
15. Simpson W.J., Ruzicka R.L., and Thomas N.R. (1974). Physiologic responses to initial dental experience. *J. Dent. Child.*, **41**, 465–70.
16. Jackson, E. (1978). Patients' perceptions of dentistry. In *Advances in behavioural research in dentistry*, (ed. P. Weinstein). University of Washington, Seattle.
17. Weinman, J. (1987). *An outline of psychology as applied to medicine*. Wright, Bristol.
18. Broome, A. (ed.) (1989). *Health psychology: processes and applications*, Ch. 1: Health beliefs and attributions. Chapman and Hall, London.

10

Fissure sealants

10.1 INTRODUCTION AND RATIONALE

Pits and fissures provide a sheltered environment in which dental plaque can develop so that these areas are particularly susceptible to dental decay. Fissure sealants are materials designed to prevent pit and fissure caries. They are applied, mainly to the occlusal surfaces of the teeth, to obliterate the occlusal fissures, thus removing the sheltered environment which favours caries progression.

10.2 HISTORICAL BACKGROUND

The problems of pit and fissure caries were recognized long ago. In the 1920s it was suggested that cavities should be prepared and filled with amalgam in all pits and fissures. This was called 'prophylactic odontotomy' and has been likened to justifying suicide with the argument that death comes to everyone sooner or later. Nevertheless, this technique was a forerunner of today's sealant.

An alternative suggestion, made in the 1960s, was that pits and fissures should be eradicated by widening them with small burs to produce rounded channels. Although more conservative than prophylactic odontotomy, this interesting idea also involved the removal of healthy tooth structure. A number of workers tried to prevent the onset of decay by applying chemicals to the fissure system such as silver nitrate, trying to make the enamel more resistant to bacterial action. Attempts were also made to occlude the fissure system with black copper cement, but both this approach and the use of silver nitrate were found to be ineffective in preventing caries.

The advent of the fissure sealants as we know them today had to wait for the development of the acid-etch technique by Buonocore in 1955. This classic work described the application of phosphoric acid to enamel, to etch the tissue, creating porosities within it. When acrylic resin was applied, the resin flowed into the holes in the enamel, thus bonding the material to the tooth. Subsequently a superior resin system was developed by Bowen at the National Bureau of Standards in America. Chemically, it is based on the product of bisphenol A and glycidyl methacrylate, commonly referred to as BIS-GMA or Bowen's resin. Most modern fissure sealants are based on Bowen's resin and are bonded to the enamel using the acid-etch technique.

10.3 THE ACID-ETCH TECHNIQUE

When 30–50 per cent phosphoric acid is applied for 60 seconds to a clean enamel surface, two things happen. First of all, a small amount of enamel is dissolved (Fig. 10.1). About 8 μm of tissue is lost, which compares with 2–3 μm lost when teeth are polished with prophylaxis paste (1000 μm = 1 mm). In addition to this loss of tissue, porosities (about 50 μm deep) are produced in the enamel surface.

Three basic types of surface characteristics have been described (Figs 10.2, 10.3, 10.4). In the most common, called type 1 etching pattern, prism core material is preferentially removed, leaving the prism peripheries relatively intact (Fig. 10.2). In the second, type 2 etching pattern, the reverse is observed. The peripheral regions of the prisms are removed preferentially, leaving prism cores remaining relatively unaffected (Fig. 10.3). In the type 3 etching pattern, there is a more haphazard effect not readily related to prism morphology (Fig. 10.4). All three etching types can be found in a single sample of etched enamel.

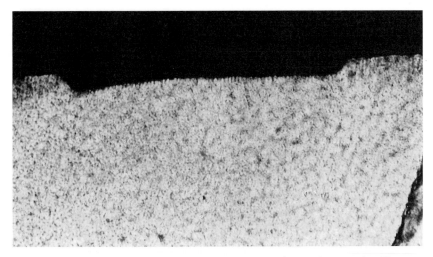

Fig. 10.1. A longitudinal ground section through an area of enamel exposed to 30 per cent phosphoric acid for 60 seconds. About 8 μm of enamel has been lost from the surface of the etched area. (Magnification ×500.)

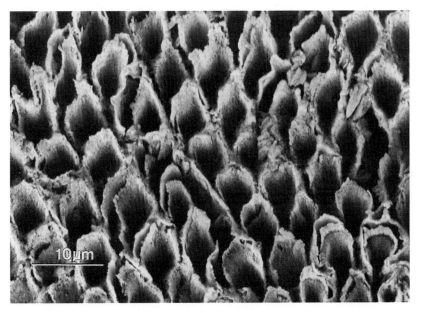

Fig. 10.2. Scanning electron micrograph of etched enamel, type 1 etching pattern. Prism core material is preferentially removed, leaving the prism periphery relatively intact. (Space bar = 10 μm.)

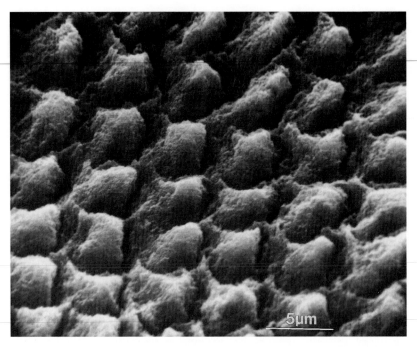

Fig. 10.3.   Scanning electron micrograph of etched enamel, type 2 etching pattern. Peripheral regions of prisms are removed preferentially, leaving prism cores relatively unaffected. (Space bar = 5 μm.)

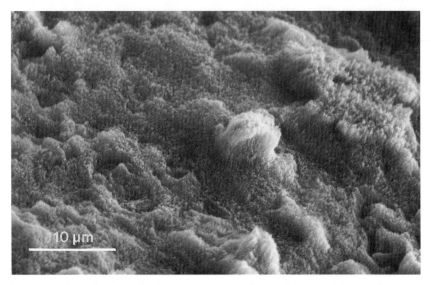

Fig. 10.4.   Scanning electron micrograph of etched enamel, type 3 etching pattern, showing a more haphazard effect not readily related to prism morphology. (Space bar = 10 μm.)

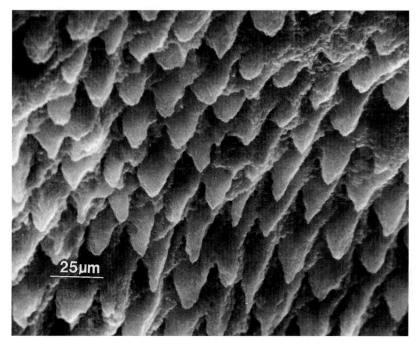

Fig. 10.5. Scanning electron micrograph of a sample of fissure sealant after demineralization of the adjacent enamel. The inner fitting surface of the resin shows tags approximately 30 μm long.

The concentration of phosphoric acid has been chosen to be between 30 and 50 per cent to minimize surface loss of tissue but maximize the depth of the porosities. Once the resin material is applied, it will flow into the porosities polymerizing to form retentive tags (Fig. 10.5).

10.4 CHOICE OF SEALANT MATERIAL

The modern fissure sealants are based on Bowen's resin. Products from many manufacturers are available giving the dentist the following choices:

1. A material cured by exposure to visible light or one that sets chemically when two components are mixed. Light-activated materials have the advantage that the operator has better control over the setting time.

2. Sealant materials may be clear, tinted, or opaque. Advocates of clear sealants claim that it is an advantage to be able to see the tooth beneath to detect any colour change that may indicate leakage and

development of a carious lesion. Tinted or opaque sealants, on the other hand, have the advantage that partial loss of the sealant is easy to see and then the sealant may be repaired.

3. Sealants are available as unfilled or semifilled resins. The latter were introduced on the assumption that the inorganic filler would improve sealant longevity by increasing the material's resistance to abrasion. While this is undoubtedly true, there is a problem of increased wear of the opposing arch which raises doubt over the use of these materials.

4. Fluoride-containing sealants are an interesting possibility, but at the moment it is not known whether resin materials will release sufficient fluoride to exert a further cariostatic effect.

10.5 CLINICAL TRIALS

Techniques and materials should be carefully investigated in clinical trials, and an enormous number of these have now been undertaken demonstrating the efficacy of fissure sealants. The materials are usually tested in the first permanent molars where they are applied shortly after eruption of the teeth.

Trials have been designed to compare fissure sealing of one molar to no treatment of the contralateral molar in the same mouth. In addition, many trials have been designed to compare different sealant materials, again in the same mouth. In all these trials retention of the sealant has been a parameter that has been carefully measured since, to be effective, the sealant must be retained on the tooth. In addition, caries status has been recorded.

The long-term results of chemically cured materials are excellent, with 50 per cent of teeth remaining completely covered after ten years. Visible light-cured sealants have not been in existence to be tested over this period, but up to an observation period of five years they appear as effective as their autopolymerizing cousins.[1]

Sealant longevity is not only influenced by the type of sealant. The position of the tooth in the mouth, the skill of the operator, the age of the child, and the eruption status of the tooth are all relevant. Thus the more anterior the tooth, the more skilled the operator, the older the child, and the more fully erupted the tooth, the better the prognosis.

10.6 CLINICAL INDICATIONS

10.6.1 Permanent teeth

Since caries in pits and fissures is difficult to diagnose in its early stage, it is logical to fissure seal susceptible teeth as soon after eruption as possible.

First and second permanent molars are obvious candidates and some dentists will decide to seal the fissures of all newly erupted permanent molars as a routine. However, this approach may be overtreatment and some of the following criteria may be useful when deciding whether or not to fissure seal[2,3]

1. How long has the tooth been in the mouth? Epidemiological studies show that lesion formation and progression may take many years in modern populations, and thus it would not be unreasonable to decide to fissure seal a molar which had been erupted for 10 years. To give an example, in a 20-year-old patient with three restored second molars, fissure sealing the questionable unrestored occlusal surface of the fourth second molar seems a logical preventive measure.

2. Can the tooth be isolated from salivary contamination? Salivary contamination during fissure sealant placement is the most common cause of failure of a sealant. With luck the sealant will fall off and there will be no permanent harm but if the sealant is partly retained and leaking, caries can progress beneath it, safe from salivary protection, fluoride ions, and detection by the dentist. For this reason good isolation from saliva is an essential part of the clinical technique with rubber dam being the most reliable isolation technique. However, in order to apply a clamp the tooth must be erupted sufficiently. Teeth can take six to twelve months to erupt sufficiently for clamp application and this is too long to wait in a high caries-risk child. In such cases a local anaesthetic and a retentive rubber dam clamp may solve the problem. Alternatively, cotton wool roll isolation and efficient aspiration could be considered. Finally, in these circumstances, consideration might be given to the use of a glass-ionomer sealant as a temporary measure (see Section 10.10).

3. Does the patient show evidence of caries in other teeth? A high caries prevalence is still the best indicator of caries risk. Caries and restorations in the deciduous dentition would favour the use of sealants in the permanent dentition. Similarly the need for restoration of a permanent molar would lead logically to sealant protection for other molars.

4. Is the patient's oral hygiene poor? Can it be improved, specifically on the occlusal surface of an erupting tooth? Such surfaces must be brushed individually, but a high degree of patient or parent compliance is required to achieve this.

5. Has the dentist reason to believe the patient's diet contains much sugar? Diet analysis is relevant when assessing caries risk and forms the basis for the individual patient's preventive regime.

6. Does the dentist anticipate that the patient may be difficult to manage when carrying out restorative dentistry? Minimally invasive procedures, like fissure sealing, may demand a little less patient cooperation. However, the technique should not be underestimated. Done properly, it may be nearly as time-consuming as a restoration and this has obvious financial implications.

7. Does the patient belong to a group where it is particularly important to prevent dental caries, for example medically compromised children, patients with cleft palates or bleeding diatheses such as haemophilia?

8. Is hidden caries present on a bitewing radiograph? Fissure sealants will sometimes inevitably be applied over early enamel lesions. However, is it safe to fissure seal apparently intact occlusal surfaces where radiographs reveal caries in dentine? Research evidence conflicts. Some workers have used microbiological and radiographic techniques to show that sealing over such lesions results in lesion arrest,[4,5] while other studies show that

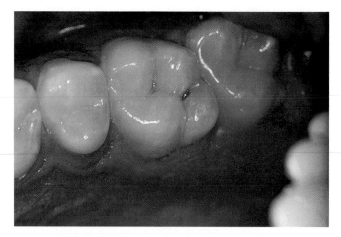

Fig. 10.6.   A deep fissure pattern that may be difficult to keep clean.

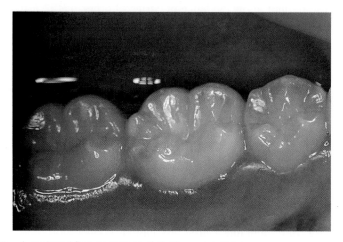

Fig. 10.7.   A coalesed fissure pattern of shallow, rounded grooves.

microorganisms may survive and flourish under sealants that are apparently intact.[6] The authors would not advocate the use of sealants over dentine caries visible on a bitewing radiograph, preferring to treat such lesions operatively with sealant restorations.

9. Does the tooth have a deep fissure pattern that will be difficult to keep clean (Fig. 10.6) or a coalesced fissure pattern of shallow rounded groves (Fig. 10.7) unlikely to decay?

10.6.2 Deciduous teeth

Deciduous molar teeth are not fissure sealed as often as permanent molar teeth. The main indication for fissure sealing is finding caries elsewhere in the dentition, i.e. caries risk is high.

10.7 CLINICAL TECHNIQUE

10.7.1 Isolation

Isolation is probably the most critical step with regard to the success or failure of the sealant. If saliva blocks the pores created by etching, the bond will be weakened. A rubber dam is the most effective method of isolation and is preferred to the use of cotton wool rolls and a saliva ejector. The latter are difficult to use because after etching the teeth must be thoroughly washed. This inevitably soaks the cotton wool rolls which must then be changed. While this is being done, it is all too easy to drop saliva over the etched tooth surface and this contamination will ruin the bond of the sealant to the enamel.

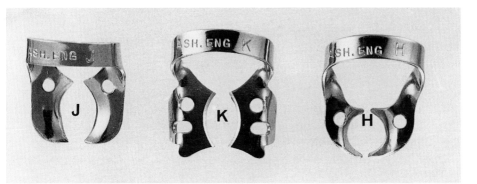

Fig. 10.8. A selection of rubber dam clamps. Clamps J and K are bland, H is retentive, J and H are wingless, K is winged.

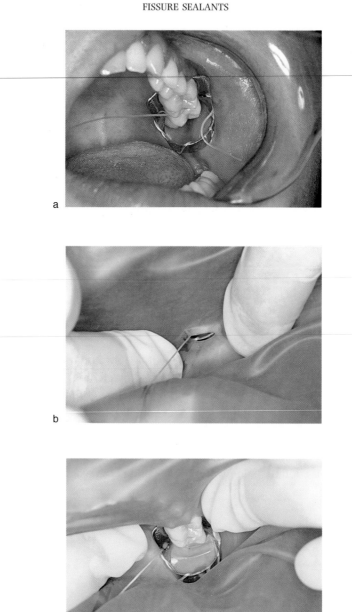

Fig. 10.9. (a) A wingless clamp in position on an upper molar. Floss has been attached to the holes of the clamp so that the dentist can retrieve it should the clamp fracture across the bow. (b) The floss is now threaded through the punched and lubricated hole in the rubber dam. (c) The dentist now slides the rubber over the bow of the clamp, one side and then the other side. The dental nurse gently pulls on the floss as the rubber is placed.

When rubber dam is applied for fissure sealing only the tooth to be treated needs to be isolated. Since a rubber dam clamp will be required, and clamps can be uncomfortable, a small amount of local anaesthetic should be infiltrated buccal to the tooth to be treated. Alternatively topical anaesthetic may be liberally applied to the gingival margin. A clamp of suitable size is selected and tried on the tooth, placing it just coronal to the gingival margin. Where the maximum convexity of the tooth is subgingival, a retentive rubber dam clamp is required, but where the tooth is fully erupted, a bland clamp should be chosen (see Fig. 10.8). Floss should be attached to the holes of the clamp so that the dentist can retrieve it should the clamp fracture across the bow (Fig. 10.9a).

If the clamp is positioned before applying the rubber, it is convenient to select a wingless clamp for molar teeth (Fig. 10.9a). Having placed the clamp on the tooth, the floss is threaded through the punched and lubricated hole in the rubber dam (Fig. 10.9b). The dental nurse now gently pulls on the floss as the dentist slides the rubber over the bow of the clamp, one side (Fig. 10.9c) and then the other side. Should the clamp fracture across the bow, the dental nurse retrieves the pieces by pulling on the floss.

An alternative technique is for the dentist to apply clamp and rubber simultaneously. In this case a winged clamp must be chosen (see Fig. 10.8) and the wings engaged in the lubricated hole (Fig. 10.10a). Clamp and rubber are applied simultaneously. The dental nurse assistant should gently retract the rubber so that the dentist can see the tooth clearly (Fig. 10.10b). A disadvantage of this method is that the dentist cannot see the gingival margin when placing the clamp. Once the clamp is in position a flat plastic instrument is used to disengage the rubber from the wings of the clamp (Fig. 10.10c). If this step is omitted, saliva will leak around the tooth.

A piece of soft material, such as paper towelling, in which a mouth-hole has been cut, is now placed between the rubber and the patient's face to prevent the uncomfortable feeling of rubber against the face. Finally the frame is positioned (Fig. 10.11).

10.7.2 Cleaning the teeth

The tooth surface to be etched and sealed must be thoroughly cleaned with a bristle brush and a pumice and water slurry. Oil-based mixtures of pumice should not be used as these may interfere with etching. The pumice is washed away with a blast of water and air from the 3-in-1 syringe and a sharp probe is dragged through the fissure system. This will remove some of the deeper plaque the brush cannot reach. The tooth is then washed again and dried thoroughly.

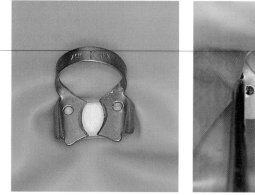
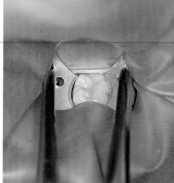

a   b

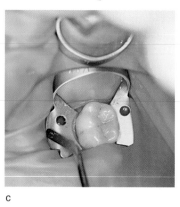

c

Fig. 10.10. (a) A winged rubber dam clamp engaged in the lubricated hole in the rubber. (b) Clamp and rubber are being placed on the tooth simultaneously. The dental nurse should gently retract the rubber so that the dentist can see the tooth clearly. (c) A flat plastic instrument is used to disengage the rubber from the wings of the clamp.

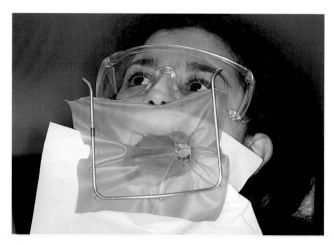

Fig. 10.11. A rubber dam in position. Note that a soft towel separates the rubber from the face. The rubber may be trimmed to avoid contact with the nose, although this was not done in this case because the patient was comfortable.

10.7.3 Etching

The phosphoric acid etchant is supplied by the manufacturer in the form of either a colourless liquid or a coloured gel. The gel is preferred as it is much easier to control. The etchant is applied over the whole occlusal surface and any lingual or buccal surface where grooves require sealing (Fig. 10.12a). Etching the entire occlusal surface avoids the danger of covering an unetched surface with sealant and thus inviting leakage. The acid can be applied with either a tiny pledget of cotton wool, a tiny gauze sponge, or a small brush. As soon as the complete area to be etched is covered with acid, the time is noted. The etching time will be given in the manufacturer's instructions and is usually 30 seconds. When acid is used in the liquid form, fresh solution can be dabbed on the surfaces during etching but care should be taken to treat the enamel surface very carefully, and not rub the cotton pellet or sponge on the surface during acid application as this may damage the fragile enamel latticework being formed.

10.7.4 Washing

After etching the acid is washed away. Initially a water spray is used from the 3-in-1 syringe to remove most of the acid. After approximately five seconds of spraying water, the air button is also pressed, forming a strong water–air spray which should be played over the etched surface for at least 15–20 seconds. If gels are used the wash time should be doubled to at least 30 seconds to ensure removal of the gel and reaction products. During the washing phase the dental nurse removes all excess water with the aspirator.

10.7.5 Drying the etched enamel

The tooth surface is now thoroughly dried with air from the 3-in-1 syringe. The drying phase is most important, since any moisture on the etched surface will hinder penetration of the resin into the enamel. A minimum of 15 seconds of drying is recommended. At this stage the etched area should appear matt and white (Fig. 10.12b). It is good practice to check that the airline is not contaminated by water or oil by blowing it at a clean glass surface. Any moisture or oil coming from the airline will cause the technique to fail.

With a rubber dam in position, there should be no danger of salivary contamination of the etched surface. If this does occur, however, it is essential to re-etch the enamel because the saliva will block the pores which are essential for optimal bonding.

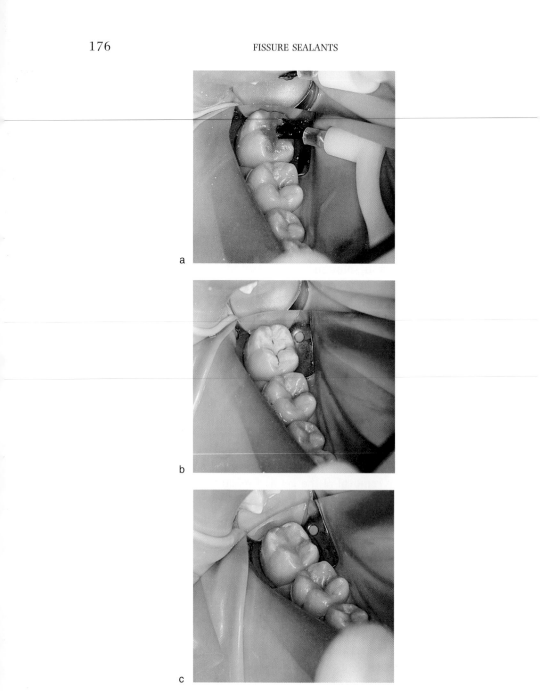

Fig. 10.12. (a) Application of the etchant gel to the occlusal surface of a lower second molar. (b) The dried etched area appears matt and white. (c) The completed fissure sealant. Note it has been applied within the etched area to ensure marginal seal. (By courtesy of Dr G. Roberts.)

10.7.6 Mixing the resin

A light-cured resin material does not require mixing. A chemically cured resin (autocuring resin) has two components which are gently mixed together to avoid incorporating air bubbles.

10.7.7 Sealant application

A small disposable brush or applicator, supplied by the manufacturer, is used to apply the sealant. The sealant is applied to the pits and fissures and up the etched cuspal slopes. If a light-cured material has been chosen, the light should be placed directly over the sealant, but should not touch it. The sealant is exposed for the full time recommended by the manufacturer to cure it. It is essential to time this carefully as an incompletely cured material is doomed to failure. In addition, with a molar tooth, the light source should be directed at the distal part of the occlusal surface for the curing time and then moved to the mesial aspect for a similar time. Any buccal or palatal groove or pit should be similarly cured with the light source directly over it.

Most chemically cured sealants polymerize in one to three minutes and the manufacturer's instructions should be consulted to check the setting time of the particular material chosen.

The outer surface layer of any sealant will not polymerize, due to the inhibiting effect of oxygen in the atmosphere. Thus the sealant will always appear to have a greasy film after polymerization (Fig. 10.12c).

10.7.8 Checking occlusion

The rubber dam is now removed and the occlusion checked with articulating paper. Whilst it is considered acceptable to allow any high spots to be abraded away when unfilled fissure sealants are used, with filled materials it is wiser to reduce high spots by grinding with a small round diamond stone in a conventional handpiece.

10.8 RECALL AND REASSESSMENT

It cannot be stressed too strongly that a fissure sealed tooth is not immune from caries. A well-bonded sealant will prevent decay but a leaking sealant is a recipe for disaster. For this reason, fissure sealed teeth must be reviewed with the same care as unfilled or restored surfaces. This means that at every recall visit the teeth must be isolated with cotton wool rolls and dried. The sealant is then checked visually. Any discoloration of the sealant, the margin of the sealant, or the underlying enamel must be viewed with suspicion as this may indicate leakage. A careful check should be made for partial or complete loss of the material. Coloured and filled resins are easier to see than the colourless and unfilled materials. However, the latter have the advantage that caries beneath them can be detected as a brown discoloration. In addition to a visual check, some operators advocate the use of a Briault probe to check that the sealant is firmly attached to the tooth and cannot be lifted off. Finally, bitewing radiographs of sealed teeth must be carefully checked for signs of caries. Operative intervention is called for if caries in dentine is seen.

A sealant which is partly lost (Fig. 10.13) or one where a margin is discoloured can be repaired by removing as much of the old sealant as possible, re-etching, and applying fresh sealant. Provided a clean surface is produced, new sealant will bond to the old material although this bond is not as strong as the original intact material.

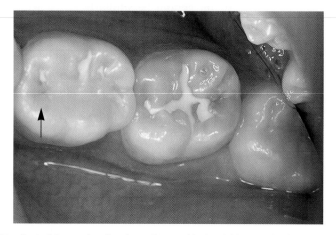

Fig. 10.13.   Part of the sealant has been lost and it should be repaired.

10.9 THE COST-EFFECTIVENESS OF SEALANTS

Some attempts have been made to assess the cost-effectiveness of sealants. If every tooth with an occlusal surface were to be fissure sealed, fissure sealing would become more expensive than the alternative approach which is the restoration of carious teeth. However, this 'blunderbuss' approach would not be a correct use for sealants because not all teeth are going to decay. Thus prescription of sealants must be based on an assessment of caries risk.

If fissure sealants were only to be used on first permanent molars, soon after eruption of these teeth, the procedure would probably be 'cost-effective'. However, if caries risk is correctly assessed, not all those teeth will need to be fissure sealed. In a population with a falling caries rate preventive efforts must be targeted at those most in need.

In addition, the value of a successful sealant must not be costed in terms of clinical time and materials alone. The technique is atraumatic in contrast to operative dentistry. On the other hand, research has shown that placing a restoration in a tooth can start a restorative cycle where restorations tend to be removed and replaced every five to ten years with a consequent increase in size of the cavity. Eventually the tooth structure is so weakened that a crown is required and a failed crown may lead to extraction.

10.10 GLASS–IONOMER CEMENTS

In recent years the use of glass–ionomer cement as a fissure sealant has been tried.[3] This material contains aluminosilicate glass and poly(alkenoic) acid and was the first permanent restorative material to be chemically adhesive to enamel and dentine. Etching of enamel is not required, but organic debris is removed using a special conditioner (polyacrylic acid) supplied with the material. This conditioning ensures a clean surface to receive the bond. An interesting feature of glass–ionomer cement is that it contains available fluoride, which may exert a cariostatic effect. In addition, the material can take up fluoride from the mouth and may thus act as a fluoride reservoir. For this reason there has been interest in the use of glass–ionomer cements as fissure sealants.

Unfortunately clinical trials show poor retention over periods as short as six to twelve months. It has been suggested that the material will only be successful in a patent fissure, where an explorer can enter, so some fissure preparation may be required if the material is to survive long term. An alternative suggestion is to use a glass–ionomer sealant as a temporary fissure sealant in an erupting tooth where isolation from saliva is a problem but caries risk demands immediate protection. The efficacy of this approach has yet to be thoroughly researched.

REFERENCES

1. Ripa, L.W. (1993). Sealants revisited: an update of the effectiveness of pit-and-fissure sealants. *Caries Res.*, **27**, (suppl. 1), 77–82.

2. A policy document on fissure sealants (1993). *Int. J. Paediat. Dent.*, **3**, 99–100.
3. Kidd, E.A.M. and Joyston-Bechal, S. (1994). Update on fissure sealants. *Dent. Update*, **21**, 323–6.
4. Handleman, S.L. (1991). Therapeutic use of sealants for incipient or early carious lesions in children and young adults. *Proc. Finn. Dent. Soc.*, **87**, 463–75.
5. Metz-Fairhurst, E.J., Schuster, G.S., Williams, J.E., and Fairhurst, C.W. (1979). Clinical progress of sealed and unsealed caries: radiographic and clinical observations. *J. Prosthet. Dent.*, **42**, 633–7.
6. Weerheijm, K.L., de Soet, J.J., van Amerongen, W.E., and de Graff, J. (1992). Sealing of occlusal caries lesions: an alternative for curative treatment? *J. Dent. Child.*, **59**, 263–8.

11

The operative management of caries

11.1 WHAT CONSTITUTES TREATMENT?

This is not a textbook of operative dentistry and readers are referred to *Pickard's manual of operative dentistry*[1] for a description of operative techniques. However, this book on caries is incomplete without some consideration of the role of operative dentistry in the management of the carious process. Practising dentists spend a major part of their time, and derive a substantial part of their income, from repairing the ravages of dental caries. Restorative dentistry is technically demanding and dental schools must devote many curriculum hours to this subject so that graduates are technically competent. Unfortunately this emphasis, although essential, has its dangers. The undergraduate may come to believe that operative dentistry is the only treatment for the carious process.

In the past dental schools may have reinforced this attitude by operating 'points systems' where points were given for operative procedures and students were signed up to take their final examination once a certain number of points had been achieved. Points were not usually awarded for preventive treatments and thus undergraduates felt that to be 'working' they must be restoring teeth. These attitudes were perhaps fuelled by the method of remuneration of dentists in the UK National Health Service. For many years dentists were paid a fee per item of reparative treatment but preventive treatments, such as dietary advice, fluoride application, oral hygiene instruction, and fissure sealing, were not individually remunerated. These attitudes were inevitably transferred to patients. Students or dentists who spent time on preventive treatments were asked by patients, 'When are you going to *do* something?' meaning, 'When are you going to place a filling?'. Thus over the years treatment of caries in adults became synonymous with operative dentistry and prevention was designated as 'the wait and watch' approach implying inactivity. On the other hand departments of children's dentistry were more enlightened.

Dental schools now teach cariology together with operative dentistry so that students can appreciate that the carious process can be modified by preventive treatment. Chapters 6–9 of this text have concentrated on these treatment techniques. They are the essential management of the carious process and are time-consuming and therefore expensive, although cost-effective in the long run. The techniques are just as worthy of remuneration as operative dentistry. Thus treatment of the carious process involves both *preventive treatment* and *operative treatment*.

Since preventive treatments demand the full cooperation of the patient it is extremely important that patients appreciate that appointments addressing plaque control, dietary advice, and use of fluoride are just as much treatment of the carious process as appointments to place restorations. Indeed, since few of us actually like having our teeth filled, a dentist whose philosophy is to help patients avoid the need for fillings will be popular!

However, high-risk patients often present requiring restorations. The dentist may find it more difficult to explain the importance of preventive treatment when the patient is experiencing discomfort and/or a cosmetic problem (Fig. 11.1a). In these cases treating the patient's problem (such as pain or an unsightly filling) is very important if the dentist is going to gain the patient's trust and cooperation in future preventive management. When discussing the importance of preventive treatment with a patient a useful analogy can be drawn with the problem presented by a building that is on fire. It would be illogical to repair the building before the flames were extinguished.

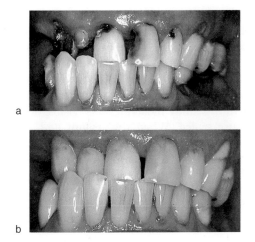

Fig. 11.1.   Before (a) and after (b) a course of treatment by an undergraduate dental student. This patient presented with a very neglected mouth and with poor motivation and low expectations of treatment. However, he has benefited not only from the student's operative treatment but also heeded the preventive advice and encouragement given. He is now highly motivated towards maintaining his remaining teeth and his whole attitude to dentistry has been changed by this experience.

11.2 WHY TREAT OPERATIVELY?

The above discussion may seem to imply that operative dentistry has only a minor role to play in the management of caries. This is not the case. There are at least 5 reasons why operative dentistry is necessary.

11.2.1 To remove infected dentine

Although the early lesion may be treated by preventive means and hopefully arrested, cavities in the dental tissues will not calcify up from the base. The cavity is a plaque trap, often inaccessible to oral hygiene aids. Once dentine is infected there may be a proliferation of bacteria and a selection for acid-producing bacteria, particularly lactobacilli. This results in the Stephan curves illustrated in Fig. 1.1 (p. 4). One aim of operative dentistry is to remove this infected dentine.

It is interesting to question this rationale by speculating whether organisms can survive, multiply, and continue the carious process if they are cut off from their source of nutrient in the mouth by a restoration. This question is unresolved but it is very important and relevant to operative dentistry. If the organisms are unable to survive without nutrients from the mouth, then fillings or fissure sealants could be placed over infected dentine. The organisms in the dentine might then die or become inactive in the carious process. There is some research evidence that fissure sealants may arrest hidden or occult fissure caries.[2,3] However, other work[4] implies that the microorganisms can survive on nutrients derived from the pulp via the dentinal tubules. In this study hidden lesions, visible only on a bitewing radiograph, were fissure sealed. When the sealant and overlying enamel were subsequently removed with a bur and the dentine sampled and cultured, considerable numbers of viable, cariogenic bacteria were found.

It is surely remarkable that such a basic and relevant question remains unanswered. The authors would suggest that at present infected dentine should be removed during cavity preparation.

11.2.2 To protect the pulp and avoid pain

In many ways operative dentistry should be considered as an exercise in protecting the pulp. One rationale for restoring a cavity in a tooth is to remove the soft, infected dentine because it is acting as an irritant to the pulp–dentine complex. Bacterial toxins cause chronic inflammation, but when the organisms actually reach the pulp (a carious exposure) acute inflammation is likely (see p. 35), resulting in pain with hot, cold, and sweet agents, which persists for minutes or hours.

Cavitated lesions may also require restoration to prevent patients experiencing pain on exposure to hot, cold, and sweet agents. Caries of enamel and dentine is not painful *per se* but loss of dental tissues, as in a cavity, deprives the pulp of insulation. Temperature sensations are partly a function of the thickness of the calcified tissues between the external environment and the pulp. Anyone who doubts this should bite into an ice cream and notice the lower incisors tingle! In addition, exposed dentinal tubules may also be sensitive to temperature and osmotic changes because of fluid movement within them. This sensitivity may gradually subside thanks to two natural defence reactions. One of these is the laying down of reparative dentine and the other is an increased mineralization at the tooth surface due to salivary action. However, in some cases restoration of the tooth is necessary to relieve pain. The restoration acts as an insulating layer between the mouth and the pulp–dentine complex.

11.2.3 To remove a source of cariogenic bacteria

Each carious cavity provide a nidus of infection where cariogenic bacteria can multiply protected from oral hygiene aids. Lactobacilli in particular flourish in stagnation areas because their growth is favoured by the aciduric conditions. Removal of infected dentine and restoration of cavities with temporary fillings is an essential part of disease control and is discussed further in Section 11.5.

11.2.4 To facilitate plaque control

Carious cavities are plaque traps often inaccessible to oral hygiene aids. Since these microbial deposits are the principal cause of dental caries the process is likely to progress. Thus a rationale behind cavity preparation and restoration must be to restore the integrity of the dental tissues by eliminating plaque traps.

The relevance of the elimination of plaque traps in operative treatment has a number of important implications. The first is that the restoration should seal the cavity and not allow leakage of bacteria between the filling and the tooth. Thus the cavity sealing ability of restorative materials is important and will be discussed further in Section 11.7.2. In addition, operative dentistry should be carried out to a high standard so that restorations and the adjacent tooth surface may be kept plaque free. Finally operative and preventive treatments must go together. Unless patients are taught to remove plaque, new carious lesions are likely to form next to the filling. Restoration of teeth would then become an expensive game of dental snakes and ladders. Restoring the cavity is the ladder but failing to improve plaque control is a potential snake because the carious process may start again.

11.2.5 To restore appearance

Carious cavities are often unsightly, especially in the front of the mouth. Patients, very understandably, are anxious to exchange a brown, discoloured hole for a tooth-coloured filling, indistinguishable from natural tooth. Indeed, one of the joys of operative dentistry is to be able to improve appearance in this way (Fig. 11.1). However, if dentists do not at the same time stress the necessity of preventive efforts, they are guilty of lulling patients into a false sense of security. Fillings do not prevent further caries. They are at best temporary in a caries-risk mouth and always a poor substitute for unblemished enamel and dentine.

11.3 WHEN TO TREAT OPERATIVELY

The rationale behind operative treatment is central to deciding when to restore. Thus operative treatment is required when infected dentine is present which may prejudice pulpal health. Restorations are also required when effective plaque control is impossible and when appearance is prejudiced. The indications for operative treatment, together with the relevant diagnostic tests, have been discussed in Chapter 4.

11.4 CARIES REMOVAL

11.4.1 Objectives of caries removal

The objectives of caries removal are:

- to remove infected dentine
- to preserve as much tooth tissue as possible commensurate with this
- to avoid unnecessary pulpal damage.

Removing infected dentine

Demineralization of dentine precedes bacterial penetration. An objective of operative treatment is to remove demineralized and infected dentine. Such dentine is soft. Research has shown that if all soft dentine is removed from the cavity, the dentine that remains is minimally infected although it will be slightly demineralized.[5] This residual demineralization would not be seen on a clinical radiograph. However, if the tooth were to be extracted so that thin sections could be cut through the prepared cavity, radiographs of these sections (microradiographs) would show a layer of radiolucent, demineralized dentine at the base of the cavity.

Preserving tooth tissue

It is important to preserve as much hard tooth tissue as possible during cavity preparation. The carious process would have inevitably weakened the tooth and the operative dentist should be anxious not to overcut the tooth as this would weaken it still further.

Avoiding pulpal damage

It is important not to damage the pulp unnecessarily during caries removal, but sometimes removal of all soft caries reveals an exposure of the pulp chamber. This is called a *carious exposure* and it is inevitable in a grossly carious tooth and important for the dentist to recognize. It implies that infection has already reached the pulp and an area of chronic inflammation will be present. Such pulpal damage is unlikely to recover and the damaged pulp should be removed and replaced with an inert filling material (a root filling).

On the other hand, removal of hard dentine may result in a pulpal exposure. This is called a *traumatic exposure* and it should not happen!

Another way in which the pulp may be damaged during caries removal is by overheating. Rotary instruments are used during cavity preparation at both high and low speed. These instruments generate heat, and the faster they rotate, the more heat they produce. Thus a water spray is used to cool high-speed rotary instruments. The student may demonstrate the potential for overheating in the phantom head room. Try cutting an extracted tooth with an air rotor without water spray in a darkened room. The bur will glow red and the dentine will smell. The pulp would be unlikely to survive such an insult if this were done in the clinic.

11.4.2 Method of caries removal

Caries removal includes the following stages:

- pre-operative assessment
- gaining access to caries
- removal of carious tissue at the enamel–dentine junction
- removal of carious tissue over the pulp.

Pre-operative assessment

The extent of the demineralization should be noted on the bitewing radiograph. The relationship of this radiolucent area to the pulp, the size of the pulp chamber, and the presence of reparative dentine should also be examined (Figs 11.2 and 11.3). Remember that a radiograph is a two-dimensional representation of a three-dimensional subject.

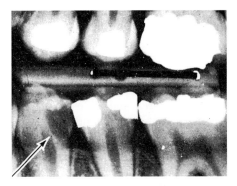

Fig. 11.2. A bitewing radiograph of a carious lesion on a lower first premolar in a young patient. Note the proximity of the lesion to the pulp chamber.

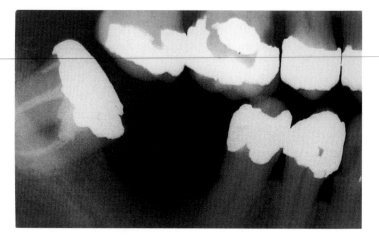

Fig. 11.3. A bitewing radiograph of a carious lesion on the mesial root surface of the upper first molar in an old patient. Note the small pulp chamber.

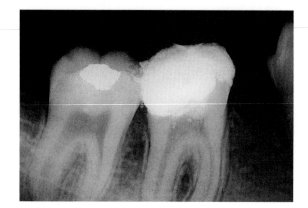
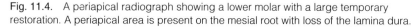

Fig. 11.4. A periapical radiograph showing a lower molar with a large temporary restoration. A periapical area is present on the mesial root with loss of the lamina dura.

A periapical radiograph should be available for teeth where a carious exposure is likely. The dentist should examine this radiograph for the continuity of the lamina dura around the apices of the teeth and any periapical area of bone resorption. A periapical area and/or loss of lamina dura imply irreversible pulpal damage. In a single-rooted tooth it is likely that no vital tissue remains in the root canal. In a multirooted tooth the root with the area will not contain vital tissue but vital tissue may be present in other root canals. These teeth require root canal treatment if they are to be saved. Thus the radiograph should be examined to decide whether this is feasible (Fig. 11.4).

Finally, a pulp test should be performed on all teeth with extensive carious lesions. Details of how this is done and the interpretation of the results are to be found in text books of operative dentistry.[1]

Gaining access to caries

On a *free smooth surface* a cavity is present in the enamel or the root surface and access to carious dentine has been made by the carious process.

On the *occlusal surface*, however, the topography of the lesion is very different because of the shape of the fissure (see Figs 3.1 and 3.2, p. 31). Thus an apparently small lesion in a fissure is often found to have undermined the enamel extensively and involve a surprisingly large zone of dentine. This enamel should be removed with an air rotor. Figures 11.5a,b show removal of enamel over a fissure lesion.

The *approximal surface* presents a rather different problem. If no adjacent tooth is present the lesion is directly accessible and the carious dentine may be approached directly through the cavity. However, a contact point is usually present and now intact enamel has to be removed over the lesion to gain access to carious dentine. The lesion may be approached by removing the marginal ridge which has been undermined by the caries and the marginal ridge is destroyed in the cutting process (Fig. 11.6).

In an attempt to preserve tooth tissue another approach has been suggested. The marginal ridge is preserved and access to caries gained by removing occlusal enamel so that carious dentine may be approached by tunnelling beneath the undermined ridge (Fig. 11.7). The preparation has been called the internal cavity preparation because access to the cavity is from within the tooth. This approach is conservative of tooth tissue but has a number of potential drawbacks. Vision and access for instruments are

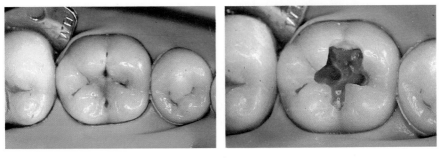

a   b

Fig. 11.5. (a) An occlusal cavity is present in the lower first molar. (b) Access to caries begins to reveal the extent of the lesion.

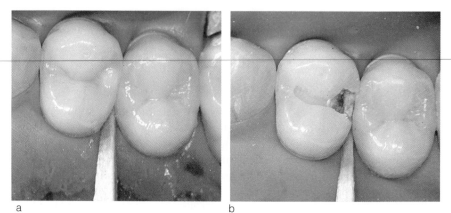

a   b

Fig. 11.6. (a) A distal cavity is present in the upper first premolar. (b) Access to caries has been gained by removing the marginal ridge.

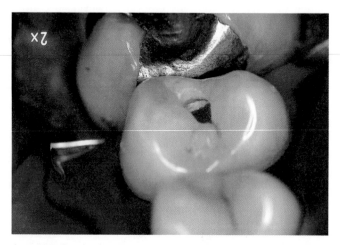

Fig. 11.7. Approximal caries has been approached from the occlusal aspect leaving the marginal ridge intact.

impaired by the marginal ridge. The carious lesion will have undermined the enamel of the marginal ridge and undermined enamel is brittle and may break under occlusal stress. However, this may not be critical because adhesive dental materials are available which may support the enamel once the tooth is restored.

An alternative access to approximal caries in posterior teeth is to approach the lesion buccally, again preserving the marginal ridge. This approach is particularly appropriate if the tooth is tilted lingually

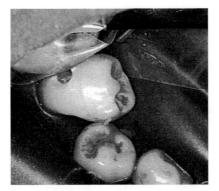

Fig. 11.8. A buccal approach to approximal caries has been used. This preserves the marginal ridge and is appropriate for this tooth because it is tilted lingually. The matrix strip will be used to contour the tooth-coloured restoration.

(Fig. 11.8) or if caries is on the root surface and thus is well away from the marginal ridge.

Access to approximal caries in anterior teeth is generally gained lingually so that the restoration will not be too visible (Fig. 11.9). Once again consideration should be given to preserving the marginal ridge. Sometimes tooth position, or the position of the lesion, may dictate a buccal approach (Fig. 11.10).

Removal of carious tissue at the enamel–dentine junction

Once sufficient access is available caries is removed from the enamel–dentine junction with round burs in the slow handpiece. Traditionally, the aim has been to remove all demineralized tissue in this area and preparation continues until the enamel–dentine junction feels hard to a sharp probe and is stain-free. However, recent research has questioned the validity of this approach since areas of the enamel–dentine junction that are

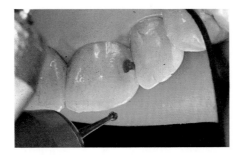

Fig. 11.9. Lingual access to approximal caries on the distal aspect of a central incisor.

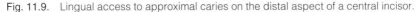

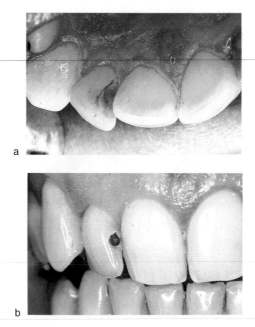

Fig. 11.10. (a) Overlapping incisor teeth with caries in the mesial surface of the lateral incisor. Access from the lingual side would be very difficult. (b) Access has been gained from the buccal surface.

hard but stained are minimally infected. Thus where tooth tissue is at a premium the authors would currently 'break the rules' and leave hard but stained dentine at the enamel–dentine junction. When cavities are prepared in areas of root dentine only soft dentine should be removed at the cavity margin. Attempts to remove all staining as well may result in very large cavities which are difficult to restore.

Removal of carious tissue over the pulp

The final stage in caries removal is to deal with the demineralized tissue over the pulp. A sharp excavator should be used to remove all soft dentine. It is unnecessary and incorrect to remove tissue that is stained but hard. To do so would invite traumatic exposure. In deep cavities the stained demineralized tissue that remains is covered with a lining material containing calcium hydroxide to encourage reparative dentine formation and kill any remaining microorganisms. This is called indirect pulp capping. It may be important to isolate a deep cavity from saliva since some research has shown that microexposures (a pulpal exposure that is too small to see) will often heal by reparative dentine formation provided that bacterial contamination is minimized. For this reason a rubber dam is useful when restoring very carious teeth.

During cavity preparation the operator must be aware that reactionary dentine will have formed beneath the carious lesion but will not be present in a part of the cavity that was not carious. In a cervical lesion the reparative dentine is more apically placed than might be expected. This is because it has formed at the pulpal end of the dentinal tubules which are running apically in this region. It is easy to expose the pulp in such cavities.

11.5 STABILIZATION OF ACTIVE DISEASE WITH TEMPORARY DRESSINGS

When a patient presents with multiple carious lesions, a combined preventive and operative approach will be required. This approach must include a careful history and examination, diagnosis of the cause of the disease, extraction of teeth which are obviously unsavable, institution of preventive measures, and stabilization of large active lesions. All lesions where pulpal involvement looks likely on a radiograph should be treated in the following way.

The tooth should initially be tested to determine whether the pulp is *vital*. If it is, a local anaesthetic is given and access gained to the carious dentine. The enamel–dentine junction is made caries-free and caries is excavated over the pulp as described in the previous section. In a vital, symptomless tooth, calcium hydroxide may be used as an indirect pulp capping agent followed by a glass–ionomer cement temporary filling.

Where caries has resulted in frank exposure of a vital pulp, removal of the pulp is often advisable to prevent pain. Eventually such teeth require root canal therapy if they are to be saved, but initially the pulp cavity may be dressed with a mild antiseptic on cotton wool and the tooth restored with a glass–ionomer cement as a temporary filling. Where inadequate anaesthesia or insufficient time preclude complete removal of the coronal and radicular pulp, a vital exposure can be dressed with a corticosteroid–antibiotic preparation before placing a temporary filling. These products are unrivalled in their ability to suppress the inflammatory process and hence the pain of pulpitis, but root canal therapy is the eventual treatment of choice if the tooth is to be saved.

Where grossly carious teeth are found to be *non-vital*, but the teeth are restorable, the pulp cavity may be dressed with a mild antiseptic on cotton wool and the tooth restored temporarily. If, however, the patient has symptoms of acute apical infection, thorough debridement of the root canal system is required before placement of a mild antiseptic dressing in the coronal pulp chamber and temporary restoration of the tooth.

Stabilization of active, advanced lesions in this way is an essential part of deciding the eventual treatment plan for the patient. It may be that some of these teeth are found to be unrestorable and their extraction will therefore be advised. It is only after such careful investigation that the dentist can estimate the extent of restorative treatment required, such as the number of root fillings. Stabilization also assists disease control by reducing infection and ensuring that toothache is not experienced in one tooth while many restorative hours are devoted to another.

In addition, during these stabilization appointments, dentist and patient will be getting to know one another. Preventive measures can be instituted and the dentist can begin to gauge the patient's attitude towards disease control in his or her own mouth. If cooperation with dietary and plaque control seems to be forthcoming, a treatment plan that preserves as many teeth as possible will be justified. If, on the other hand, the patient appears uninterested and disinclined to play their essential role in disease control, a treatment involving some extractions and simple restorations may have more chance of success in the long run.

Definitive restorations should not be started in such a patient until prevention has been instituted and grossly carious teeth stabilized.

11.6 FAILURE OF RESTORATIONS[1,6]

Restorations commonly fail in one of two ways: new disease or technical failures. New disease includes new caries, either around a restoration (recurrent or secondary caries (Fig. 11.11)) or at another site on the tooth, tooth wear, pulpal problems, and periodontal disease. Restorations may also fail as a result of trauma. Technical failures include fractured restorations, marginal breakdown, and fracture of cusps adjacent to restorations. Defective restoration contour, for instance a deficient contact point, an over-hanging margin, or occlusal degradation and wear of a filling, will also cause dentists to replace restorations. Finally, if the filling becomes loose or drops out it will need replacing. Poor appearance may also trigger the decision to replace a restoration. Many, but not all, technical failures may be objectively diagnosed clinically. Marginal breakdown and discoloration of the filling material are examples of subjective judgements which may or may not lead to replacement, depending on the clinician. Recurrent caries also leads to difficult and often subjective diagnoses.

Defining the reason for failure is important if future failure is to be avoided. For instance, if new caries is the cause of failure, preventive treat-

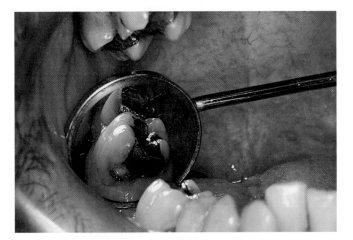

Fig. 11.11.   A cavitated carious lesion is present at the cervical margin of the restoration in this molar.

ment demanding patient cooperation is also required. Such patient-based factors are often the most difficult to influence. On the other hand, technical failures may be more under the operator's control and some of these failures occur as a direct result of a shortcoming in the restorative technique. In such cases, changing the technique or the material used may make future success more likely.

Some causes of failure of restorations are of particular importance because replacement fillings are so common. Surveys on the reasons for replacement of restorations in general practice will be reviewed to set the subject of recurrent caries in the context of overall failure.

11.6.1 Surveys on the reasons for replacement

A number of cross-sectional and longitudinal studies have been carried out in general dental practices to see why dentists replace restorations. Several points of practical importance surface from these surveys. Only three or four different diagnoses covered 80–90 per cent of all reasons for replacement (Fig. 11.12).

The clinical diagnosis of recurrent caries was by far the most common reason for replacement of amalgam and composite restorations. Glass–ionomer cements, on the other hand, were less likely to fail in this way and this may be due to the available fluoride in the material exerting a cariostatic effect.

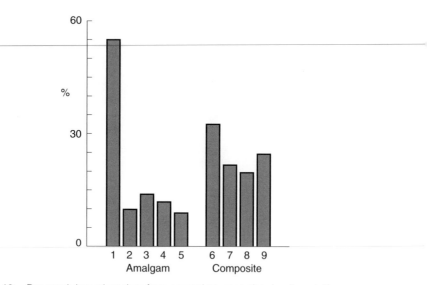

Fig. 11.12. Bar graph based on data from several sources showing the relative proportions of reasons for failure of amalgam and composite restorations. 1: recurrent caries; 2: marginal degradation; 3: isthmus fracture; 4: fracture of tooth; 5: other reasons; 6: recurrent caries; 7: discolouration; 8: poor anatomic form; 9: other reasons. (By courtesy of the *International Dental Journal*.[6])

11.7 RECURRENT CARIES

Since recurrent caries is such an important reason for dentists replacing restorations it is important to consider the histopathology of the lesion, the relevance of the quality of the restorative material, and how recurrent caries should be diagnosed.

11.7.1 Histological features of recurrent caries

Histological examination of the early recurrent or secondary carious lesion gives some indication of how such a lesion is formed (Figs 11.13 and 11.14). When a filling is placed, the adjacent enamel may be considered in two planes—the surface enamel and the enamel of the cavity wall. For this reason, a secondary carious lesion has been described as occurring in two parts—an 'outer lesion' formed on the surface of the tooth as a result of primary attack and a cavity 'wall lesion' which will only be seen if there is leakage of bacteria, fluids, molecules, or hydrogen ions between the restoration and the cavity wall. This clinically undetectable leakage around restorations is referred to as 'microleakage'.

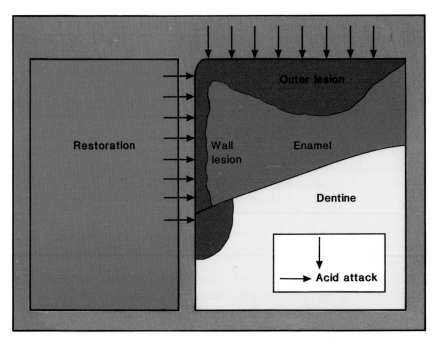

Fig. 11.13. A diagrammatic representation of recurrent caries showing that the carious lesion may occur in two parts: an 'outer lesion' formed on the surface of the tooth as a result of primary attack and a 'cavity wall lesion' formed as a result of leakage between the restoration and the cavity wall.

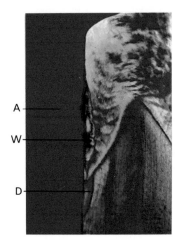

Fig. 11.14. Longitudinal ground section of a recurrent carious lesion. The ground section is in quinoline and viewed with polarized light. An occlusal amalgam restoration was present but lost during section preparation (A). The wall lesion is seen as a dark zone (W). Dentine involvement is obvious (D). There is an outer lesion in this case.

11.7.2 Microleakage and the relevance of the wall lesion

Many techniques have been devised over the last 25 years to test the cavity sealing properties of restorations both in the laboratory and in the mouth. These include the use of dyes, radioactive isotopes, air pressure, bacteria, neutron activation analysis, scanning electron microscopy, and artificial caries.

Essentially this vast volume of experimental work has shown that all currently available restorative materials leak to some extent. This means that if the carious challenge continues, all currently available restorative materials will fail eventually, although some will fail more quickly than others! Thus fillings do not prevent new disease and restorative care must be combined with preventive treatment.

The relative importance of the outer and wall lesions in recurrent caries is not clear, and consideration of individual filling materials and sites where caries may occur is relevant.

Although the freshly packed amalgam restoration leaks, with time the seal improves as corrosion products from the amalgam block the microspace between the filling and the tooth. When extracted teeth with amalgam restorations that have been present in the mouth for some time are sectioned, wall lesions are frequently found (Fig. 11.14). However, it is likely that these lesions formed within a few weeks of the filling being placed during an initial period of leakage and that the carious process then arrested. Surveys of dentists' decisions to replace restorations show that most amalgam restorations fail approximally. This is the area where plaque will be most difficult to remove. It must be suggested, therefore, that with a well condensed amalgam restoration recurrent caries is new primary caries next to the filling. In other words the outer lesion is of prime importance.

Composite resin restorations also provide a good seal where sufficient acid-etched enamel is present. However, the gingival aspect of a composite restoration can be a problem because here the cavity margin may be either thin enamel or dentine only. Unfortunately composite resins shrink as they polymerize and then move away from the gingival margin towards the stronger bond with the enamel on the axial aspects of the cavity. Neither the use of dentine bonding agents nor glass–ionomer cements will predictably prevent this leakage, although the situation can be improved by specific handling techniques such as incremental packing and light-reflecting wedges.

However, there is still the possibility of a large gap (in bacterial terms) between filling and tooth on the cervical aspect of a composite restoration. The wall lesion may have more clinical relevance in this situation. However, the cervical aspect of the tooth is difficult to keep clean without daily flossing and thus an outer lesion may form next to the filling. Surveys of dentists' decisions to replace fillings show that recurrent caries is most often diagnosed on the cervical and approximal aspect of a restoration, the area where plaque stagnation is most likely.

Glass–ionomer cements are interesting restorative materials as far as caries is concerned. These materials contain and release fluoride. They can also take up fluoride from the mouth and may therefore be regarded as fluoride reservoirs. Since availability of the fluoride ion at the point of acid attack delays lesion progression, these restorations should be more resistant to the development of recurrent caries than most materials.

All cemented restorations (inlays and crowns) rely on the cement lute for their cavity-sealing ability. A laboratory study has shown that cements can leak, but once again the relevance of wall lesion formation is unknown.

11.7.3 Diagnosis of recurrent caries

As with primary caries, the dentist needs good lighting, dry clean teeth, sharp eyes, and good bitewing radiographs. A sharp probe may be useful to clear plaque from a tooth surface but the probe should not be jammed in between the filling and the tooth as it may cause damage.

Sharp eyes

What visual signs are there of recurrent caries and how should these appearances be managed? A white or brown spot lesion around a restoration (Fig. 2.2, p. 21) should be noted and managed by preventive treatment. A cavitated lesion adjacent to a restoration (an outer lesion) (Fig. 11.11) should be treated operatively as well as preventively when the lesion is a plaque trap.

A particular problem with amalgam restorations is marginal breakdown or fracture, often called 'ditching' (Fig. 11.15). This has long been regarded with suspicion by clinicians. The appearance has been considered synomous with recurrent caries and the restorations replaced as a preventive procedure to avoid plaque stagnation in this area. However, there are now a number of reasons why this approach is both incorrect and unnecessarily destructive. First of all ditching normally occurs occlusally whereas most recurrent caries occurs approximally and cervically. It seems unlikely, therefore, that ditching predisposes to recurrent caries. In addition laboratory studies have shown a poor correlation between caries prevalence and marginal defects. A clinical study that related ditching to the level of infection of dentine once the filling was removed showed that only ditches wide enough to admit the tip of a periodontal probe (over 0.4 mm) were associated with significant infection of the dentine. Where such a wide ditch is

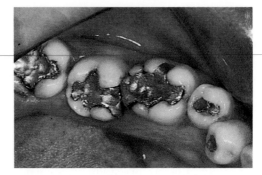

Fig. 11.15. Ditched amalgam restorations.

present it is suggested that initially this area is repaired and the whole restoration only removed if clinical evidence of active caries (soft dentine) is found. Finally research has shown that dentists may overcut cavities when removing fillings. Occlusal cavities may increase in size by as much as 0.6 mm. The dentist may perpetuate the error of cavity preparation and restoration which caused the ditching problem. This is often too sharp an amalgam-margin angle which makes the edge of the filling prone to fracture.[7] The tooth is thus in danger of entering a repetitive restorative cycle until the dentist literally runs out of tooth tissue.

Discoloration around a restoration with clinically intact margins is very difficult to interpret (Fig. 11.16). With amalgam a grey or blue discol-

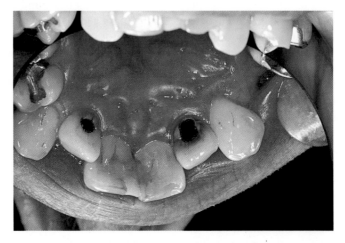

Fig. 11.16. The enamel around the amalgam restorations on the palatal aspect of the upper lateral incisors is discoloured. Is this discoloration due to caries or corrosion of the amalgam? A decision was made to replace these restorations and removal of the amalgam revealed discoloured, *hard*, dentine.

oration may indicate demineralized stained dentine, corrosion products from the amalgam or may simply be caused by light reflecting from the amalgam itself through the relatively translucent enamel. A clinical study has related stain around amalgams to the infectivity of the dentine once the filling is removed. Results showed no difference in infectivity of the dentine when stained and unstained margins were compared, provided that the margin was clinically intact or slightly ditched. This study suggested that staining may represent residual caries left when the cavity was originally prepared, which subsequently picked up exogenous stain from the mouth as a result of leakage. The authors therefore suggest that staining around an amalgam restoration should not trigger its replacement unless a carious cavity or very wide ditch is also present (Fig. 11.11).

Colour changes around tooth-coloured filling materials come in a number of forms. A white or brown spot lesion may be present and preventive treatment is indicated. The development of a line of stain at the junction of the filling and the tooth probably indicates leakage (Fig. 11.17). A laboratory study has shown that these restorations are more likely to show wall lesions than unstained margins. The authors would suggest preventive treatment unless the patient requests replacement of the filling because of poor appearance.

Stain around a tooth-coloured filling can also present as grey or brown discoloured dentine shining up through intact enamel (Fig. 11.18). It would seem likely that this appearance may represent residual caries left when the cavity was originally prepared. Alternatively it may represent active caries as a result of leakage. It is not possible to distinguish between them clinically, which is unfortunate because active caries would benefit

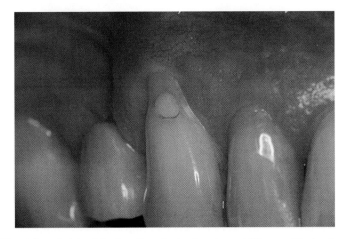

Fig. 11.17.   A line of stain at the junction of a tooth-coloured filling and the tooth.

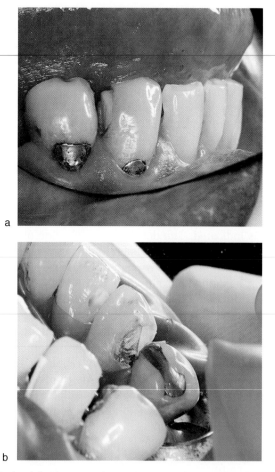

Fig. 11.18. (a) Stained dentine around a tooth-coloured restoration. (b) The appearance of the cavity once the restoration had been removed. Stained and demineralized dentine can be seen.

from restorative treatment while residual caries would not! We suggest that at present such restorations should be replaced.

Bitewing radiographs

Bitewing radiographs are of great importance in the diagnosis of recurrent caries. However, it may not always be possible to distinguish new caries from residual caries left when the restoration was placed. Nevertheless, radiolucent areas are likely to be infected and the restorations (Fig. 11.19) should be replaced.

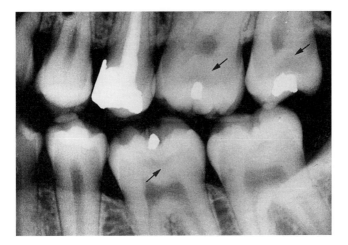

Fig. 11.19.   A bitewing radiograph of very small occlusal amalgam restorations with caries in dentine showing as radiolucent areas (arrows). It is not known whether this represents residual or recurrent caries but these restorations should be replaced because such radiolucent areas are usually heavily infected.

Since recurrent caries usually occurs cervically, careful examination of bitewing radiographs is very important in diagnosis. It follows, therefore, that restorative materials should be opaque. Figures 11.3 and 11.20 show radiolucent areas next to the cervical margins of amalgam restorations. This is infected dentine and the fillings should be replaced. These are likely to represent new lesions that have formed in areas of plaque stagnation next to the fillings. New restorations are indicated but preventive treatment is also very important if the lesions are not to recur. Figure 11.21 shows a bitewing radiograph of an amalgam restoration in a lower first molar with areas of radiodense dentine beneath the restoration. This appearance represents residual

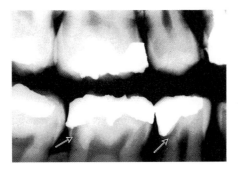

Fig. 11.20.   A bitewing radiograph showing root caries cervical to amalgam restorations. New restorations are indicated but preventive treatment is also very important.

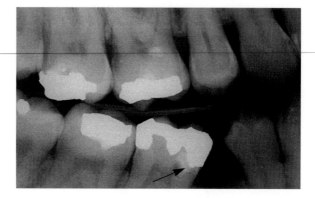

Fig. 11.21.   A large amalgam restoration is present in the lower first molar and areas of radiodense dentine are present beneath the approximal aspects of the filling. These areas probably represent residual demineralized dentine left when the cavity was originally prepared. Tin and zinc ions from the amalgam have passed into these areas to give the radiodense appearance.

demineralized dentine left when the filling was originally placed. Tin and zinc from the amalgam have passed into the demineralized area to give the radiodense appearance.[8] The authors would not replace this restoration.

11.7.4 Auditing the decision to treat operatively

The diagnosis of recurrent caries is not clear cut. One consequence of this is that dentists will not agree on when restorations should be replaced. The dental student will know this, having seen different teachers arrive at different treatment plans for the same tooth. One teacher may insist the filling is replaced. Another may suggest reviewing it in six months, while a third may not note any abnormality. Figure 11.22 is typical of a restoration where dentists may not agree on whether it should be replaced. However, dentists and dental students can audit their clinical decisions when fillings are replaced. If the decision to operate is correct, soft dentine should be found when the filling is removed. Each decision to replace a restoration can be audited in this way.

11.7.5 Patient education and review

Clinicians who have not seen some of their work fail over the years are either myopic, dental gods, or very young. The most beautiful restorative work will fail in the caries-prone mouth if further disease is not prevented.

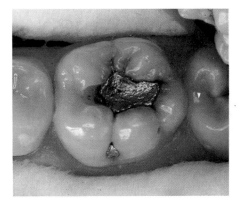

Fig. 11.22. Would you replace this restoration?

Attempts should be made to find out whether the advice given on diet is being followed and consideration should be given as to whether some form of topical fluoride, such as a mouthrinse, should be continued. Oral hygiene instruction needs reinforcement, and this is particularly important where Class II restorations, crowns, or bridges are present. Frequent review is advisable in the caries-prone mouth to reinforce prevention and check the restorations.

REFERENCES

1. Kidd, E.A.M. and Smith, B.G.N. (1995). *Pickard's Manual of Operative Dentistry*, (7th edn) Oxford Medical Publications, Oxford.
2. Handleman, S.L., Leverett, D.H., Espelando, M.A., and Curzon, J.A. (1986). Clinical radiographic evaluation of sealed carious and sound tooth surfaces. *J. Am. Dent. Assoc*, **113**, 751–4.
3. Mertz-Fairhurst, E.J., Schuster, G.S., and Fairhurst, C.W. (1986). Arresting caries by sealants: results of clinical study. *J. Am. Dent. Assoc.*, **112**, 194–7.
4. Weerheijm, K.L., de Soet, J.J., van Amerongen, W.E., and de Graaff, J. (1992). Sealing of occlusal caries lesions; an alternative for curative treatment? *J. Dent. Child.*, **59**, 263–8.
5. Kidd, E.A.M., Joyston-Bechal, S., and Beighton, D. (1993). Microbiological validation of assessments of caries activity during cavity preparation. *Caries Res.*, **27**, 402–8.
6. Kidd, E.A.M., Toffenetti, F., and Mjör, I.A. (1992). Secondary caries. *Int. Dent. J.*, **42**, 127–38.
7. Elderton, R.J. (1984). Cavo-surface angles, amalgam-margin angles and occlusal cavity preparations. *Br. Dent. J.*, **156**, 319–24.
8. Rudolphy, M.P., van Amerongen, J.P., and ten Cate J.M. (1994). Radiopacities in dentine under amalgam restorations. *Caries Res.*, **28**, 240–5.

Index